HOMEOPATHIC
MEDICINE
FOR WOMEN

Homeopathic Medicine

for Women

An Alternative Approach to Gynecological Health Care

TREVOR SMITH, M.D.

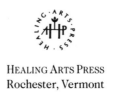

HEALING ARTS PRESS
Rochester, Vermont

Healing Arts Press
One Park Street
Rochester, Vermont 05767

Library of Congress Cataloging-in-Publication Data

Smith, Trevor, 1934-
  Homeopathic medicine for women : an alternative approach to gynecological health care / by Trevor Smith.
    p.   cm.
  Rev. ed. of: A woman's guide to homeopathic medicine. 1984.
  Includes index.
  ISBN 0-89281-236-2 (pbk.)
  1. Generative organs, Female—Diseases—Homeopathic treatment.
2. Genito-urinary organs—Diseases—Homeopathic treatment.
3. Women—Diseases—Homeopathic treatment. I. Smith, Trevor, 1934-
Woman's guide to homeopathic medicine. II. Title.
RX465.S65 1988
618--dc19   88-23536
                                          CIP

Printed and bound in the United States

10 9 8 7 6 5 4

Healing Arts Press is a division of Inner Traditions International, Ltd.

Distributed to the book trade in Canada by Book Center, Inc.,
      Montreal, Quebec
Distributed to the health food trade in Canada by Alive Books,
      Toronto and Vancouver

CONTENTS

The author expresses grateful thanks to Mr Ian Donaldson F.R.C.S., F.R.C.O.G., friend and colleague, for his support, help and interest in the preparation of this book.

INTRODUCTION

It may seem a little odd for a homoeopathic doctor to be writing about gynaecological problems in the nineteen-eighties. It is an area where surgery and the latest advances in medicine and diagnostic techniques are important, and frequently used for both investigation and treatment. In a speciality using such sophisticated methods, and one in which such tremendous technical advances have been made over the past decade, it would seem that homoeopathy could at best play only a very limited role.

Women experience the field of gynaecology in different ways. For some it is the routine annual 'pap' cervical smear test where microscopic techniques can reveal pre-cancerous cellular changes at a very early stage. For others it is the convenience of the contraceptive pill, the 'copper seven' IUD or the diaphragm. Yet other women see their gynaecologist for the opposite reason — because of infertility. For them, the 'fertility pill' and the reality of the test-tube baby have brought renewed hope.

Much real and tangible progress has been made, but however real and exciting the advances in the early diagnosis and investigation of gynaecological problems, there are several reasons for being cautious about these advances.

Perhaps inevitably, the media and the popular imagination have glamorized the progress because it has been so dramatic, but in many areas of gynaecology progress is still slow and often specialized, leaving possible solutions to many problems still at an experimental level, with little practical application for the patient in the foreseeable future.

It is also becoming increasingly clear that many of our modern drugs, including the oral contraceptive and the fertility pill, can be dangerous for the patient. In many cases their risks outweigh their apparent advantages, and such powerful and indiscriminate drugs can no longer be prescribed lightly. Many modern treatments, especially the hormonal ones, have now been found to be positively dangerous to many parts of the body, and they are often potentially carcinogenic. The health risks to women can be high when neither physician nor patient fully realize at the time that the treatment is still largely experimental, and therefore a potential hazard.

An important loss to the woman patient in recent years is that the individual approach to her as a person is becoming increasingly rare. The quality of caring for the individual woman is being progressively eroded as individual attention and counselling become less and less part of the art and skill of medicine and increasing attention is given to laboratory reports and technicians. In many ways the art of diagnosis and cure has been preserved and appreciated more by gynaecologists than in other specialities, as they tend to stay more human than many of their colleagues, and retained an understanding of the woman's overall needs. They have often become more like the family general advisor because of their sensitivity to the psychological as well as the physical needs of their patients, but all too often this attention has been severely lacking and many patients have been subjected to unnecessary operations because of an overall policy rather than a strict necessity.

Many gynaecologists are now having second thoughts about the 'wonder' drugs produced by the pharmaceutical industry, and are becoming as concerned as their patients about the possible long-term effects of certain hormonal treatments. As far as the individual patient is concerned, it is still the quality of individual caring and understanding, the personality and sensitivity of the doctor, and the art of listening and communication which are most important and most appreciated. Iatrogenic disease, or doctor-induced illness, has become increasingly common, and it is vitally important for all doctors to remember that if they cannot offer much help for an individual problem, they should at least do their utmost to avoid making the patient worse by their prescribing. In many cases the results of treatment just do not match the expectations of advanced surgery and diagnostic techniques. Unless a gynaecological condition gives a clear-cut indication for surgery, the results are often far from successful, and can be disappointing for a variety of reasons. In such very frequent problem areas, like menstrual irregularity, menopausal discomfort or infertility, after all the sophisticated investigations, the outcome of treatment is often inconclusive. It is particularly in these more general areas that homoeopathy has a real role to play as a positive alternative which does not put the patient at risk.

Homoeopathy is based on old and well-proven traditions of treating 'like with like', or a remedy which produces very similar symptoms to those which the patient already experiences. The two groups of symptoms — those of the remedy and of the patient — are matched. Although it appears to have nothing new or scientific to offer in the field of gynaecology, homoeopathy does contribute a great deal to the relief of symptoms and to the needs of the patient.

Whatever the limitations of homoeopathy, it never makes the patient worse. It is often at the stage when repeated conventional treatments are failing or causing intolerable side effects that the homoeopath is consulted. All too often the hot flushes, the drenching sweats, the discharge or rash is just not improving, and the patient has increasing doubts as to the wisdom of yet more complicated prescriptions or further investigations which do nothing other than to leave the patient increasingly ill, desperate and depressed.

Many patients are told that there is nothing really wrong with them if the investigations come back negative, and are told that they must learn to live with their condition — as if it doesn't exist as long as the electronic machinery can throw up nothing as a diagnosis.

In a technological age where machinery, computers and gadgetry have already to some extent taken over from the sensitivity and intuition of doctors, the patient is ignored more and more, and becomes little more than a cog in a diagnostic machine of investigations and specialized reports. As medicine becomes increasingly sophisticated and computerized it becomes more remote and inhuman. The great danger is that as doctors increasingly become technicians, they are also more and more removed from the art of medicine and sensitivity to the needs, fears and feelings of the patient, and their own intuitive knowledge.

Almost without exception, every patient has had some experience of a bad or allergic reaction to a prescribed drug. Inevitably this leads to a shattering of the often fragile doctor-patient relationship, and the patient is offered yet another 'new' drug to counteract the side-effects which is often nothing more than a slightly altered antibiotic, tranquillizer or steroid.

However great the technical advances, the patient still needs to know what they are putting inside their body and why; the advantages, success rates and risks involved. The many and frequent side effects of the method need more explanation and often more caution, the patient should be more informed of the early signs of danger when prescribed hormonal replacement, steroids, symptomatic or contraceptive treatments, whatever their strength or form.

In certain age-groups and hereditary patterns, there is a real risk of an increased incidence of circulatory disease or cancer, which every woman should know and be fully aware of. This is no scare story; it is reality, and patients need to know more of the facts in order to assess the advantages and risks in a balanced, non-pressurized and well informed way for themselves.

Every woman can benefit from learning to trust her instincts and feelings. She must be able to ask questions like: 'Is it absolutely necessary to have this operation and what will happen if I do nothing about it now?'; and 'Do I really have to have this growth removed?' It is important not to go along passively with every surgical decision. Surgeons are human, and it may just be more convenient for a particular bias, opinion or approach to operate. If you don't mind a scar or an operation and don't want to take any risk at all, then there is no problem, but if you do care about remaining 'intact' and don't want to be scarred or operated upon unless absolutely vital and really necessary, then you must be at times prepared to do battle and ask 'Is my operation really necessary?'

For a variety of reasons — partly of the doctors own making and partly due to lack of time and pressure of work — such essential information is insufficiently given, if at all. But the patient is often also to blame, and lack of healthy pressure from patients, of demand, and of intelligent and pointed questions over the years, allows doctors to become woolly in their thinking, and to prescribe by convenience and habit when they should be intelligently assessing each prescription according to the needs of the individual patient. All too often the patients are left in the dark about what they are taking and left to their own worst fears and doubts as to diagnosis, because they fear intruding upon the doctor's time with 'silly and trivial questions' which is vital to their peace of mind. They often fear making the doctor angry — which is not at all uncommon in some practices — or are afraid of being thought foolish or neurotic and labelled as such in the doctor's notes. Such fears can very easily lead to a break in the essential confidence between patient and doctor, and undermine communication and early diagnosis.

Many unhealthy attitudes still linger from the past, when there was far too much emphasis on a form of misplaced moral purity which led to shame and delay in seeking a proper and early gynaecological diagnosis. A discharge, a rash, even self-examination, was felt to be unclean and a thing of shame and criticism. These attitudes have been present for a very long time, and only recently have things started to change significantly, but progress in these areas is difficult and inevitably slow because of the psychological depths concerned for each individual woman and scars of pressures from the past. All too often these attitudes have been unconsciously carried over into the present day. Only in very recent years has there been something of a revolution, with a new generation of more sensitive and informed women and men emerging, more free and much less restricted by out-moded concepts of their bodies. They are daring to challenge the old taboos and ideas so that a more healthy attitude and the real prospect of earlier diagnosis is occuring. I now see daily in my practise such people, who are easily recognizable by their questions and attitudes, and who are characteristically very alive in the real way that they relate to their doctor.

The modern woman, however well-informed, needs to know more about the workings of her body, including modern theories and ideas about how she can remain healthy, and the causes and prevention of disease. Where a treatment is envisaged, she needs to know the advantages and risks of a particular method. Almost certainly she will have read magazine articles outlining the advantages and limitations of different treatments, yet however well-informed, she will always have important questions in need of clarification, and these need to be discussed as early as possible with her doctor. When the doctor also uses homoeopathic remedies, as is increasingly common, she will want to know both about the homoeopathic approach and her doctor's conventional thinking. Every woman should clearly ascertain from her doctor, whatever his or her orientation, whether a second opinion is desirable at any stage in her gynaecological treatment, especially if a favourable response is not forthcoming from the doctor she first consults.

It is fundamental to homoeopathy that the whole condition of the patient be explored during the consultation, and that all relevant experiences and areas of confusion, fear and doubt be given an airing and discussed fully. This is not only vital within homoeopathy, it is basic to any medicine if it is to be human and sensitive. Every consultation leads on to a variety of other thoughts and questions which need some time for clarification and discussion, physical examination and reassurance. The patient may want to ask for explanation in a particular area, either because they are confused or anxious, or because they are not sure that they have expressed themselves adequately and clearly. Whatever the reasons given, they are always important and should be taken seriously for the patient's well-being and early diagnosis and prevention.

It is now becoming increasingly recognized by both medical profession and patients, that many female conditions are perfectly well and adequately treated by the homoeopathic method. It will combine perfectly well with other allopathic conventional treatments when these are required, except where the conventional drugs being used are primarily suppressants; in this case homoeopathy is contra-indicated and in general ineffective.

Why Homoeopathy?
The reasons for considering homoeopathy in the treatment of gynaecological problems are threefold.

1. Totality of Approach
Every female illness must be considered from the point of view of both the female hormonal cycle and the emotional factors. The two are inseperable and can profoundly affect each other. It is well known that physical cycles can and do effect the emotions, and this overall approach is important in the consulting room, where the patient must be free to choose her particular form of self-expression and approach to the doctor, be able to ask questions, and to be listened to.

　She needs her fears to be taken seriously, as much as her physical symptoms. This listening, feed-back and attention to detail, however unnecessary it may seem, is very important in homoeopathic diagnosis, and has been fundamental to its totality of approach ever since its formulation by Hahnemann two hundred years ago, and is basic to its attitudes and principles.

2. A First-line Approach in Gynaecological Problems
Homoeopathy is an important primary treatment for many gynaecological problems which do not have a direct mechanical cause, or are predominantly surgical in their treatment. It is especially useful in such problems as irregular, missed or painful periods, difficulties at the menopause, and where infection or infertility is not due to obstruction. The common uterine and bladder weaknesses of the older woman, where strain and multiple pregnancies have taken their toll, can also be relieved.

3. A Secondary Supportive Treatment
Whenever there is a problem that is basically mechanical and surgical in its treatment and diagnosis, with a physical problem that must be corrected, adjusted, removed or repaired, such as a growth that is suspect or potentially invasive, then the treatment is surgery. In every case, however, it is vital to the patient that the diagnosis, treatment and after-care be fully discussed and understood by the patient and family beforehand, with plenty of time

allowed for a full discussion of any underlying confusion, fears, doubts, or for any questions that need clearing up. All of this makes the patient more relaxed, confident and trusting, thus ensuring a better outcome from the operation, fewer complications afterwards, and a minimal recovery time.

The Female Cycle

Healthy sexual functioning is one of the most important aspects of a woman's life, as well as the most personal and intimate. It is particularly important during the reproductive years, but hardly less so at puberty or after the menopause, when body awareness and health are of major significance.

The cyclical nature of female sexuality has taken many years to escape from the slur of impurity which led to so many taboos surrounding menstruation. A revolution in thinking and attitudes has at last led many women out of the bondage of soiled and often 'dirty' self-imagery, but it has been a long process, and many negative feelings still remain.

Such cycles are a basic and essential part of female sexuality, and inseperable from all that is female in terms of depth, intuition and sensitivity. They contribute to a woman's wisdom, since each month she is very deeply aware of how life is being recreated and prepared at so many different levels within her. Only women can experience such awareness of their glandular and physiological functioning, with a clear sense of build-up to the cycle, a knowledge of retention to be followed by one of flow, which affects her whole life at every level. Ovulation is very commonly experienced quite consciously, and is often associated with a surge of sexual feelings.

After the flow there is a sense of relief and relaxation from tension for most women as the hormonal and glandular discharges have reached their peak levels and then declined. Every human being is basically a cyclical creature with a complicated system of inter-related body clocks, timetables, ebbs and flows, functionings and body levels, yet only a woman can be consciously aware of the depths of change. In a man, such changes are inaccessible because all his rhythmic changes, including the male menopausal ones, have become lost to consciousness in the remote past, together with a great deal of intuition and sensitivity, which is far more strongly retained and developed in women.

These physiological cycles are a close link between body and mind. When a period is upset, delayed or absent, it can provoke profound feelings of anxiety, restlessness and deprivation, because it is so much a part of her overall being. In a similar way, an acute emotional stress can commonly inhibit ovulation, delay the next period, or make for irregularity. The sperm-count in men can also fall dramatically to very low levels when he is under emotional pressure.

It is now strongly suspected that chronic stress or repressed emotion may be important causes in many of our more serious and common 'diseases of civilization', including cancer. If this proves true, then it is likely that it is the inhibition of healthy hypothalamic functioning within the mid-brain — intimately connected with the organization and physiological control of uterine and ovarian functioning, which is at the centre of the problem. Certainly the many patterns of modern living which are alien from anything rhythmic or natural must pass through the important nerve centre of the hypothalamus. Much of the problem is that more and more of these patterns are accepted as normal, and are no longer sensed in any way as detrimental or abnormal.

Society matures in direct proportion to the growth and maturation of its individuals. This is true both emotionally and physically. As the old habits of misunderstanding and judging the menstruating woman are finally being overcome, the modern woman can relate more healthily to her own body and its functioning. She can take a much more active and positive role in prevention of disease by regular self-examination and check-ups as she is more able to accept herself without shame.

Nevertheless the process of maturation, openness and communication is still painfully slow, particularly within the specializations of the medical profession. Obtaining any sort of diagnosis or information is often extremely difficult. The defensive and hierarchical structure of division and sub-division, of allocating different bits of the patient into different units and sections, is still the general rule. The care of and responsibility for the patient is often lost in the division of medicine into sub-specialities, and it is impossible to get any adequate facts at all about diagnosis or treatment without creating a fuss. Doctors outside the speciality often fare no better than the patients or relatives when seeking information, or trying to contact the physician with overall responsibility for the patient.

All of this is changing but often too slowly. At last patients are learning to ask questions, daring to make more demands from the doctor or specialist, requesting another opinion and asking about alternatives to a proposed operation or course of treatment. The patient now wants to know whether a more watchful and conservative approach to a problem is not just as safe as surgery. They now want to be sure that an operation is not just recommended for cosmetic reasons or the tidying up of statistics.

To lose a womb, or to have an abortion or an ectopic pregnancy, is always a psychological trauma to some degree, even if it is well-hidden or denied. Too often such grief around a surgical loss is denied at the time, pushed underground, only to emerge sometimes many years later. At the time of the operation, feelings are usually denied and suppressed out of supposed consideration for the medical process, and the family. In a hysterectomy ward feelings are particularly out of place, because this part of your anatomy is supposed to be trivial and insignificant, and without psychological importance.

The sensitive woman is not afraid of listening to or showing her emotions and feelings. She does not fear being contradictory or going against the system. Nor is she afraid of appearing to be difficult — after all she knows it is *her* body which is threatened by the scalpel. She is able to accept decisions but needs to be informed and to know the facts. When she knows all the possibilities — however frightening or upsetting — she can accept an inevitable operation or treatment without overwhelming anxiety because she understands why it is needed. What *no* woman ever wants is to be treated as a number on a list or in a ward.

Unless the patient herself takes the initiative and the trouble to ask questions, then often nobody else will do it for her, and she risks falling into a general and overall formula which may not be at all what she herself is wanting. Always ask questions, however difficult and daunting it may seem and no matter how unpopular you make yourself. These are your rights as a patient and intelligent human being. Have the strength and the courage to act whenever your intuition and sensitivity tell you.

Menstruation

The monthly cycle is essentially a process of renewal, during which the ovum develops, matures and releases itself. Not only does the cycle involve evolution and expansion into perfection and readiness for possible fertilization, but with a supreme example of nature's anticipation and preparation, it provides an embedding mechanism and food storage to nourish the already-dividing embryonic cells from the first days onward. This preparation process involves the lining layers of the uterus, together with those of the vagina, cervix and fallopian tubes, all linked in a cyclical pattern of harmonious change. There is an intelligence at work here, whereby the glands and the cells know immediately whether there has been a successful ovulation or the beginning of a pregnancy; and these events can often be sensed by the woman herself within a few hours of their occurence.

Menstruation is under the control of both local and remote hormonal triggers. At the ovarian level there are two key hormones — oestrogen and progesterone — responsible for the development of the uterine endometrial lining. At a central level are the pituitary and hypothalamic triggers and control systems, responsible for ovulation. The anterior pituitary, triggered by the hypothalamus, is responsible for the production and secretion of the two major controlling hormones — follicle-stimulating and luteinizing. Follicle-stimulating hormone — FSH — is responsible for the proliferation of follicle cells around the developing ovum and its eventual release at ovulation. These follicle cells are very important because they are the source of oestrogen from the fourth day of the cycle onwards, stimulating the replacement and thickening of endometrium and the development of related changes in the fallopian tubes, vaginal lining cells and in the cervical mucous plug which guards the entrance to the uterus. The other central control is luteinizing hormone, LH, released to a very high level to trigger off ovulation when oestrogen levels reach a critical point on approximately the fourteenth day of the cycle.

At this point the mature ovum is released into the fallopian tube and the follicle-cell remnants re-organize themselves to form a new site of hormonal release known as the corpus luteum. This is significant because from the eighth to tenth day of the cycle it is the major site of progesterone release. If the ovum fails to be fertilized no chorionic gonadotrophins are produced to give the signal for the continued development and retention of the corpus luteum, so it degenerates and progesterone levels fall sharply. This acts as a trigger for a new cycle of menstruation to re-commence. The actual period occurs as the endometrial surface layer of the uterus is sloughed-off ready for replacement and renewal of a new potential embedding area. Bleeding, discharge and drainage of the uterine cellular matter takes place, including of course the microscopic unfertilized ovum of the previous cycle.

The Role and Action of Oestrogen

Oestrogen is produced from the fourth day of the cycle by the new maturing follicle cells of the ovary, under the stimulus of pituitary FSH. Its major action is on the endometrial uterine lining, thickening the cellular layers so that the straight glandular cells develop with a high sugar or glycogen food and energy content. At the same time there is increase in the cellular sodium or salt content in the area. Specific changes also occur within the cervical mucous plug at the uterine entrance and within the vaginal lining layers. Increased salt build-up makes some degree of water-retention inevitable, and may be a cause of early cycle swelling and discomfort. As the cycle progresses, everything is organized for the imminent ovulation since if fertilization occurs it leaves little time for delay — the process of division starts immediately, and food and energy must be there waiting. Already some 100 cells have been formed by the time of embedding in the uterus.

The effects of oestrogen are widespread, and many women are well aware of them reaching peak levels because the glands and duct cells of the breasts are stimulated, and there may be swelling and tenderness. Both vaginal and cervical cellular layers are also affected by oestrogen build-up, and vaginal mucous discharge may increase at this time of the cycle. There are many tests to ascertain whether ovulation is occurring. The ferning (which, when dried, has a fern-like appearance) test is one frequently used, whereby the increased sodium content of the cervical mucus is used to decide whether the woman is predominantly in an oestrogen phase. The elasticity of cervical mucus is often employed as a test of ovulation. It is very stretchy at this time. The fallopian tubes and the movements of the hair-like fimbrial fringe gently guide the ovum down the tube are under oestrogen influence, ensuring optimum tube positioning at the moment of ovulation. The contraction of these muscles and ligaments may sometimes cause discomfort just prior to ovulation, and when the contractions become particularly strong at ovulation, some women may experience cramping until the second half of the cycle has commenced and oestrogen dominence is less marked.

The Role and Action of Progesterone

Progesterone is produced from the remains of the ruptured ovarian follicle cells which contained the developing ovum before it was extruded into the fallopian channel. Progesterone is essential for the development of the second half of the menstrual cycle. It is produced at the same time as oestrogen, which continues to be secreted in a balanced relationship with progesterone. A different secretory phase of the cycle starts once ovulation has occurred, with well-marked characteristics clearly differentiated from the pre-ovulatory follicular phase. Unless there is a mechanical failure or obstruction, the presence of progesterone indicates fertility, ovulation and ovum release. Under the influence of progesterone, the endometrial lining cells become more twisted and complex, no longer the simple, straight tubes of the oestrogen phase. There is a marked increase in blood supply as well as an increase in sugars and basic enzymes, and the salt content decreases. Often this increased vascularization causes breast discomfort; the breasts become heavier, swollen and tender because of glandular proliferation and because of the increased fluid volume in preparation for lactation should the ovum be fertilized.

Progesterone also acts on the vaginal mucous cell lining, producing a decrease of superficial cells and enhanced growth of the intermediate cells or middle layers. This can be clearly seen in a vaginal smear test taken at this time. A further change indicating that ovulation has occurred is that the cervical mucous plug becomes thinner, more alkaline and easily penetrable, forming an ideal environment for the young sperm. With increasing progesterone build-up the mucus changes again and becomes thick, more acid, and more of a sperm barrier than a supporting medium. Progesterone output continues for about nine or ten days after ovulation, and then as the corpus luteum begins to degenerate, the levels fall significantly on about the twenty-fourth day.

There is a fall in both oestrogen and progesterone levels at this time, with the declining ovarian hormonal levels acting as the trigger for menstruation on the twenty-eighth day. It is during the last few days of very low oestrogen and progesterone output that premenstrual changes often occur, with many of the characteristic emotional and physical symptoms. With bleeding, the entire endometrial layer of cells is sloughed away. Bleeding occurs intermittently, usually with a maximum loss on the first day. Menstrual loss is variable throughout life, with an average of twelve ounces for the full period.

All the phases of the cycle are dependent upon healthy hypothalamic and putuitary functioning. Because the pituitary is situated in an enclosed, saddle-shaped area within the skull, the least external pressure from a nearby swelling, such as an aneurysm or adenoma, can interfere with its functioning. This is why, when there is menstrual irregularity, it is often common practise to X-ray the skull to look for signs of possible pituitary displacement.

The vagina plays a crucial role in reproduction, and its layers are intimately involved in the whole menstrual cycle. Embryo-embedding occurs in the uterus, but the vagina acts as the vital pathway for fertilization, and in this role must be optimally conducive to sperm survival and motility. As well as its role as the exit canal for the monthly cast-off uterine layers, it is also the natural channel for the foetus and afterbirth during childbirth.

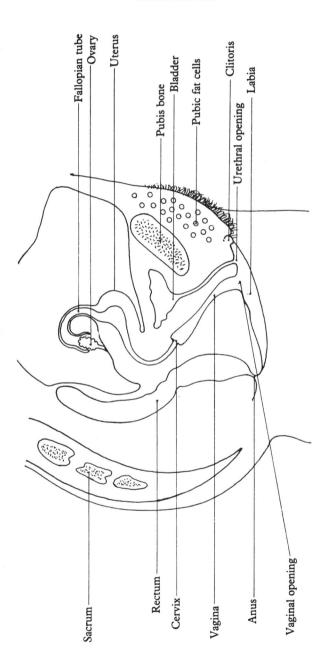

Basic female anatomy (diagramatic).

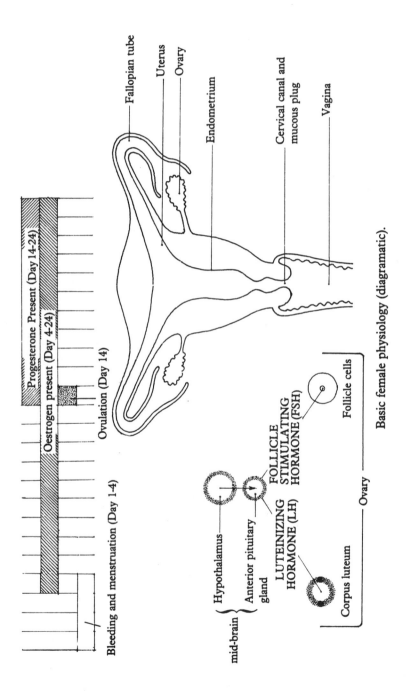

Basic female physiology (diagramatic).

1.

ADOLESCENT PERIOD
PROBLEMS

Adolescent girls often suffer both physical and emotional discomfort during the early menstrual years. Their periods are frequently short, painful and irregular, and a regular cycle may take many years to become established. These discomforts are an unwelcome addition to the many other emotional problems of the teenage years, when shyness, doubts and uncertainties about sexuality can sometimes be quite severe.

Adolescence is a time of exploration and discovery. It is also a time of experimentation, especially sexually, and this sometimes leads to an overindulgence in smoking, alcohol, junk foods, pop music, television, promiscuity, drugs, and sometimes crime. Sexually transmitted diseases are all on the increase, and 'fashion' often means wearing inappropriate clothes. All of this puts pressure on an adolescent frame, and inhibits healthy ovarian growth and function when in excess. It is not uncommon to see teenagers who seem old, worn-out and cynical before they have barely lived. They have been exposed to drugs, alcohol and tobacco, and often to an appalling diet, as well as frequently a disturbed emotional, and sometimes violent, background. It is not surprising that such children often seem to remain curiously immature, and alongside a weak pattern of general health, they tend to suffer from period problems. This is fortunately not widespread, but to some extent all adolescents are under pressure, at an age when they need the greatest guidance and support.

Delayed Onset of the Menstrual Cycle (Primary Amenorrhoea)
All girls are concerned about when they will have their first period because they know that it means the onset of their adult sexuality — what it will

feel like and how painful it will be. Unless a girl has been completely uninformed about her periods so that they come as a shock to her, an extremely rare situation in our present society, she is nearly always anxiously waiting for them to manifest, especially since other girls in her class will have made it known when they have started. The age of onset is very variable, but is occurring at a younger age than ever before as diet and nutrition improve. With each successive generation, physical maturity arrives earlier and earlier. The commonest age of onset for most girls is from twelve to thirteen, but the range is between ten and seventeen. Most physicians would only make a diagnosis of delayed onset if periods have not begun by a girl's seventeenth birthday. This failure of menstruation to appear is sometimes called primary amenorrhoea, to differentiate it from the absense of periods after a time when they have been established.

Causes of Primary Amenorrhoea

Inherited or constitutional genetic reasons are the commonest cause, the delay being due to a factor which is absent so that the gonads or ovaries fail to mature. The follicle cells do not proliferate and oestrogen is not produced. Immaturity may be at a genital gonadal level, or at the level of pituitary function, often for unknown reasons. Physical causes are rare, but obesity, perhaps associated with a pituitary abnormality such as Cushing's disease or thyroid disease, can be a contributory cause. These conditions not only inhibit growth and energy and the burning of food and fat within the body, but ovarian development is also depressed and sometimes non-existent.

Hormonal and endocrinal causes of primary amenorrhoea include failure of the ovaries to function or the inhibition of normal ovarian development and maturation due to pituitary disease. Physical obstructions and blockages are very rare causes. An imperforate hymen may obstruct the blood flow, and rarely a congenital or birth defect of the vagina, uterus or ovaries causes interference with normal functioning.

Shock in any form, especially psychological shock, can cause a profound delay in the onset of menstrual functioning. Psychological reasons for delayed menstruation include such common and profound problems as anorexia nervosa, severe depression, schizophrenia, and Down's syndrome (mongolism).

Symptoms of Primary Amenorrhoea

In most cases there are no other symptoms than that the menstrual flow fails to start; otherwise the secondary sexual characteristics are normal. In a few cases the breasts are underdeveloped and small, and pubic hair is thin or minimal. Often the girl seems physically ready, but is unusually late. In some of these cases both mother and grandmother had a late onset, and the process is determined purely by hereditary factors.

Recommended Remedies for Primary Amenorrhoea

1) Pulsatilla
One of the best and most useful remedies, especially when the girl is immature, moody or easily tearful, with a passive temperament. There are often a variety of accompanying symptoms, especially palpitation or nausea. In spite of a general chilliness, there is almost total intolerance of heat in any form.

2) Sepia
This remedy is a classic one, and has been used successfully by many homoeopaths. The major indication is a thin leucorrhoeal discharge due to long-standing vaginitis in a pale, thin and exhausted girl with depressive solitary tendencies and sometimes extreme irritability. The skin is often sallow with a yellowish tinge to it, and dragging lower abdominal pains are sometimes present.

3) Bryonia
This is a valuable remedy for the more flushed, constipated girl without anaemia or pallor, often with a constant dry cough and periodic loss of blood from other areas, such as monthly nose bleeds.

4) Calcarea
For the sluggish, chilly and rather fat girl, always pale and late in her milestones since birth. Colicky pains, headaches and dizziness are common, and there is often a peculiar intolerance of any form of tight clothing. She is nearly always tired and lacks energy as well as warmth.

5) Kali. carb.
These girls are usually well-built and of nervous disposition. Chronic catarrhal symptoms are common, together with left sided lower abdominal and back pains. Palpitations, fear, and anxiety at being left alone are all frequent. In general the colicky pains are worse in the early night hours, around 3 a.m.

6) *Graphites*

The girl is often depressive in mood, and complains of sharp lower abdominal pains. The skin is nearly always affected — typically with a weeping eczema behind the ears. General health is poor, with chilliness, rheumatic pains, and hand or joint swelling.

Secondary Amenorrhoea

This differs entirely from primary amenorrhoea in that the menstrual cycle has already begun and become established, but then ceased either abruptly or slowly, and there is now an absence of ovulation. The adolescent has matured sufficiently to initiate the cycle, but the monthly cycle has not continued.

Causes of Secondary Amenorrhoea

All too often the causes are not clear, and have to be a matter of conjecture. Most gynaecologists would be reluctant to subject a young woman to a battery of tests and investigations without waiting to see whether the cycle will spontaneously re-commence.

Pregnancy is the commonest cause of secondary amenorrhoea in all ages of sexually mature women. Any sudden and severe shock to the system can also cause the condition. The shock may be physical or psychological, varying from a traumatic assault to a road-accident, a sudden loss of a close member of the family to anorexia nervosa, severe depression, or the use of addictive drugs.

Constant physical agitation can upset the normal delicate hormonal balance so that there is a failure to ovulate and produce the normal cycle. Athletes and long-distance marathon joggers may not ovulate and experience a normal cycle during long periods of training. Constant travel, such as that experienced by air hostesses, can also affect the cycle. Secondary amenorrhoea is also common as a side reaction to certain drugs, especially the steroid suppressants, and can also be the result of stopping taking the contraceptive pill.

Symptoms of Secondary Amenorrhoea

The menstrual cycle fails to occur, with an absence of the normal associated secondary sensations of breast and ankle heaviness or fluid retention.

The Conventional Treatment of Secondary Amenorrhoea

There are no clear-cut guidelines as to what to do, and many gynaecologists are wisely conservative when faced with this condition, preferring to wait and see. Some will attempt a hormonal replacement therapy, and progesterone is often tried. My own opinion is to try and avoid any hormonal replacement or stimulant therapies whenever possible, especially for younger women, unless there is true indication of a lack of hormones which has been confirmed by the laboratory. In general that sort of confirmation is extremely rare. If secondary amenorrhoea persists into the late teens it may be a cause of infertility in an early marriage. In this case Clomiphine (Clomid) is often used to stimulate ovarian functioning.

Recommended Remedies for Secondary Amenorrhoea

1) Aconitum

Recommended when the loss is the result of any sudden exposure to chill or fright. It is best taken as soon as possible after the period has been missed, but it can also be effective when a severe fright occurred in the even remote past. Headache, restlessness, aggravation by heat, a red face, thirst and general mood of irritability are common. Palpitations are often caused by the general sense of apprehension and oppression.

2) Belladonna

In many ways this remedy resembles the indications for Aconitum without the previous exposure to an emotional trauma. Typically the girl is red-faced and flushed, thirsty with frequent nose-bleeds due to the general state of congestion. There may be a mood of restless excitement or irritability.

3) Sulphur

Useful for fairly long-standing cases of unknown cause with diarrhoea, skin itching, excessive insatiable hunger and leucorrhoea. Weeping is frequent, and sometimes irritation.

4) Ignatia

Of value when the periods have been suppressed due to grief or loss.

5) Calc. carb.

The typical symptoms here are chilliness and weakness, often with forehead sweating and colicky pains with fatigue and exhaustion. The legs feel heavy and tired, and there is intolerance of any weight from the clothes or tight-fitting garments.

6) *Lycopodium*
When the periods have ceased in a sensitive, intellectual girl after exposure to an acute emotion. Right sided low abdominal pains are often present.

7) *Opium*
Where the periods have ceased for an unknown reason and the girl is excessively tired and exhausted or prone to fainting and falling asleep. Both face and head feel heavy.

8) *Platina*
Useful when there is a combination of constipation, lower abdominal colic and anxious restlessness. The disposition must be somewhat proud and haughty for the remedy to be properly indicated.

9) *Sabina*
Consider this remedy when the periods have been suppressed for unknown reasons, and the girl has a leucorrhoeal discharge due to a vaginitis infection.

10) *Pulsatilla*
Consider pulsatilla when there has been a sudden stoppage of the menstrual pattern after exposure to damp, especially wet feet.

Painful Adolescent Menstruation
Menstruation is painful with lower abdominal cramping pains, sometimes also felt in the lower back and kidney regions. Usually the pains are limited in their duration, and tend to occur on the day of the period's onset, or pre-menstrually on the day before the onset of bleeding.

Causes of Painful Adolescent Menstruation
In general these are largely unknown, and in most cases are put down to immaturity of hormonal function and hormonal imbalance. The present accepted theory is one of hormonal insufficiency, probably at an oestrogen level, but its exact cause is unknown. In some cases the symptoms may be psychologically induced. A recent theory concerns a newly discovered group of hormones called prostaglandins, which occur throughout the body and are now increasingly being shown to be essential to normal functioning. When present in excess they are thought to cause cramping pains, and this excessive build-up is believed by some authorities to cause contraction of the uterus and period pains.

Symptoms of Painful Adolescent Menstruation

Pain and cramping discomfort are the main symptoms, usually causing some degree of incapacity and interference with normal living. The pain usually occurs on the first or second day of the period, which may itself be weak, irregular and infrequent — sometimes as much as every six or seven weeks, so that the girl is never sure of her dates, often only the cramping pains heralding the onset of the next period.

The Conventional Treatment of Painful Adolescent Menstruation

The allopathic approach is hampered by the causes of painful menstruation being so little understood. In many cases the approach seems to be one of trial and error, and often pain-killers such as the aspirin type of analgesics or codeines are used. In the past pethidine was used extensively until it was realized how very dangerous it is, with the very considerable risks of addiction which more than outweigh its medical advantages. The oral contraceptive pill is often prescribed in an attempt to stabilize the periods, and to correct hormonal imbalance. Similarly a newly developed anti-prostaglandin group of drugs is frequently prescribed, with very mixed results, because the method is at present largely experimental and theoretical.

Recommended Remedies for Painful Adolescent Menstruation

1) Pulsatilla

This remedy is useful and nearly always prescribed at some time during treatment. It acts best when well indicated with variable colicky and tearing pains, often in the lower back or kidney regions. The menstrual loss is usually only slight, and nausea or vomiting often accompany the pains, typically accompanied by floods of tears.

2) Belladonna

The pains are more generalized and stitch-like, and begin before the period starts. Dragging heavy pains in the lower abdomen are typical, the face is hot and flushed, and the mood one of anger and irritation.

3) Chamomilla

This remedy is indicated where the pains are very severe and colicky, and associated with restlessness. Diarrhoea, irritability and fainting are common features.

4) Mag. phos.
There are spasms of cramp-like severe pains in the lower abdomen and uterus, usually relieved by warmth and movement.

5) Coffea
Severe colicky pains are present, often disturbing rest and sleep with cramp-like pains, mainly in the lower abdomen, causing distention. The pains are often described as being of a turning, twisting type. Vulval irritation is not uncommon.

6) Nux vom.
This remedy is indicated by constipation and cramping spasms of pain. The girl is easily moved to anger, and sometimes to violence. The periods are nearly always early, protracted and exhausting.

7) Sulphur
Another very useful and often prescribed remedy. Heat is a common symptom, with hot burning pains, a red face, and frequent nose-bleeds. In general the periods are early and often pale in colour. Untidiness and disorganization are the general rule. Hunger is often marked, and some form of skin infection or eczema is frequently present.

Irregular Adolescent Periods
The periods are irregular, and a regular cycle is not established. It is important to realize when considering this problem that irregularity can be quite normal, and the healthy adolescent will often menstruate on a twenty-one day cycle, or can have cycles as long as five or even seven weeks until her late teens or even later.

Causes of Irregular Adolescent Periods
In many cases the causes are unknown. The girl has never established a regular cycle, but is healthy and strong in all other respects. The causes which are most often evoked are hormonal imbalance and lack of oestrogen output, but the hormonal theories are mainly empirical.

Symptoms of Irregular Adolescent Periods
Usually periods are either missed or absent, and then recur without any regular pattern or cycle. Pain is often absent. The adolescent never knows exactly where she is in her cycle, and often little or no warning is given before

sudden bleeding occurs. Sometimes there may be slight spotting on the day of the expected onset and little more. Most commonly the period is delayed for up to two weeks and then there is a normal period, to be followed by another cycle of irregularity and delay.

The Conventional Treatment of Irregular Adolescent Periods
This is often not very satisfactory — various hormonal replacement therapies are often tried including the oral contraceptive pill, but the success is rarely very encouraging.

Recommended Remedies for Irregular Adolescent Periods

1) Pulsatilla
One of the most useful remedies when the periods are at all variable, delayed or late. The pulsatilla characteristic of chilliness with intolerance of heat and excessive emotional display is usually present in a girl with a passive disposition.

2) Dulcamara
This remedy should be used when the periods are often late and the flow is thin, pale and short-lasted.

3) Ferrum met.
Usually indicated for the thin, anaemic, rather flushed girl, who is nearly always exhausted and whose periods are frequently late.

4) Sulphur
This is a remedy for a girl with a combination of late periods, and the typical sulphur temperament of constipation, hunger, itchy skin and frequent flashes of heat.

5) Sepia
This is sometimes indicated when periods are delayed and accompanied by a combination of severe and exhausting dragging pains and a tendency to faint.

6) Carbo veg.
The menstrual flow is nearly always early and heavy with colicy pains preceding or accompanying the flow. Toothache or an itchy skin may precede

the onset of the period. Flatulence and exhaustion are common.

7) Platina
The periods are usually early, the loss thick and often dark. The intestines feel dragged down into the vagina, causing considerable discomfort. The attitude to others is always one of superiority.

8) Phosphorus
The periods are early and the loss heavy, with typical colicky pains, restless irritability, and sometimes flashes of heat. The girl is in general very nervous and often needs considerable reassurance.

9) Mag. carb.
There is a scanty flow and the periods are usually late. Nausea and extreme hunger are characteristic.

10) Natrum mur.
The periods are often early, protracted and heavy. The girls is usually tired, the skin sallow, slightly shiny and damp, with an earthy discolouration. She is often very weepy and emotional.

11) Graphites
In general the periods are delayed and late, and often there is an irritating itchy pruritus present in the vulval region.

2.

PERIOD PROBLEMS OF
THE ADULT WOMAN

Irregular Periods

The common adult problem of irregular and unstable periods, unpredictable dates and cycle patterns, affects many women. The normal cycle varies between twenty-five and thirty-three days, and few women have a precise twenty-eight-day cycle. What is important in menstrual irregularity is the variation from the normal length of cycle rather than the absolute length of the cycle. As long as the woman knows where she is with her own pattern, then all is well.

Causes of Irregular Periods

The causes are usually unknown, and in most cases are assumed to be due to hormonal imbalance within the progesterone/oestrogen cycle. Progesterone levels in particular are suspected of being at fault.

The Conventional Treatment of Irregular Periods

Hormone replacement therapy is often used, with the aim of dampening down the assumed high progesterone levels by giving additional oestrogens. This method is fraught with dangers, because of the interference with normal hypothalamic and pituitary functioning. All hormone adjustment and replacement therapies should also be treated with caution and suspicion by women because of the possible cancer risks.

Recommended Remedies for Irregular Periods

The periods are too short and bleeding occurs early

1) Ambra grisea
The period occurs early with a heavy flow, and is associated with severe pruritus vulvae and often stitch-like lower abdominal pains and a thick white discharge. Most symptoms are worsened by lying down. There is often a haemorrhagic discharge between periods, precipitated by the least pressure.

2) Carbo veg.
The periods are heavy and early, and associated with very severe lower abdominal cramping pains. An itchy skin is a typical indication, especially when colic and low backache occur after the period. Vomiting and toothache have also been reported as indications.

3) Ipecacuanha
The periods are heavy, bright red and early, followed by extreme prostration and weakness.

4) Nux. vom.
The periods are always irregular and unreliable, often early, heavy and prolonged. Spasms of lower abdominal cramping pain are common from the first day. The usual mood is one of irritability and anger.

5) Sabina
Periods are heavy, prolonged and early, associated with labour-like colicky pains and often with clotting. Often the period stops, starts again, and then just as abruptly ceases.

The periods are delayed

1) Causticum
Severe menstrual colicky pains are associated with a delayed brief period, usually only present during the daytime with no loss during the night hours.

2) Conium
The period is always late, or absent altogether. The loss is small lasting a day or two at most. Itching pruritus of the vulval area is often present, and is an indication for the remedy.

3) Dulcamara
There is a tendency for the periods to be delayed or totally absent, especially in cold and damp weather. In general the periods are short, scanty and pale.

4) Graphites
Severe colicky pains accompany a weak, short, pale, delayed period. Often associated with a depressive mood and pruritus vulvae.

5) Lachesis
Severe colic in the lower abdomen or sometimes the left ovary. The periods are delayed and brief, with a dark, thick loss, often with clots. Most symptoms are aggravated in the morning and after sleep. Restlessness and depression are both common.

6) Pulsatilla
The periods are always very variable and unpredictable, but often late and colicy, the loss dark but varying with each period, the bleeding stopping and then starting again with no fixed pattern. Nausea and palpitations are common.

7) Sepia
The periods are late and light, associated with a dragging low backache, colicky pains and exhaustion. Uterine cramps before the period are also common. There is a sense of the uterus prolapsing, and a feeling that it should be pushed back or prevented from falling further. Irritability and desire for rest and solitude are marked.

The periods are irregular and short

1) Alumina
The period is short-lasting, sometimes early, with a pale flow, and typically followed by weakness or collapse and headache. Colicky pains and headache may occur. Constipation is usually marked and severe.

2) Baryta carb.
Brief, weak periods, often associated with infertility and reduced breast development. There is often a thick white leucorrhoea which is usually worse in the week preceding the onset of the period.

3) Conium

The periods are often late, and nearly always short or almost absent. Pruritus vulvae is typically associated, and often painful low abdominal spasms. The breasts are often tender and fibrocystic, sometimes feeling stoney and hard.

4) Kali. carb.

The periods are always irregular, often diminished, and without much colour. Both before and after the flow has begun there is often pain in the kidney regions, and a feeling of pressure and weight in the uterine area. The vagina is very tender and oversensitive.

5) Pulsatilla

A useful remedy when the periods are brief but thick, with a dark, almost black, loss, often with clots.

Dysmenorrhoea (Painful Periods)

Regular pain may occur either before or at the onset of bleeding, and in some cases it may occur throughout the period, although this is fairly unusual. A severe case may involve pain and discomfort to the point of being incapacitated for fifteen days of the cycle. Dysmenorrhoea is often grouped into spasmodic and congestive types. The spasmodic type is associated with cramping lower abdominal pains beginning at the onset of bleeding, and lasting for up to seven or ten days. Congestive dysmenorrhoea is different, being more of a dull ache beginning just before the period, and disappearing as soon as bleeding starts.

Causes of Dysmenorrhoea

The causes are often unknown, and dysmenorrhoea is usually put down to hormonal imbalance. There are many theories, and the excessive action of the corpus luteum is often considered to be a fault. Excess prostaglandins are thought to be a possible cause, with excessive Prostaglandin F_{2a} a prime candidate, increasing progesterone build-up from within the uterine lining layers, provoking uterine contractions and cramps. Hormonal imbalance and hormonal instability have also been implicated, causing the endometrial lining to become excessively thick, later coming away in large fragments during the period. The pain is usually considered to be from spasm of the uterine walls. Emotion is often a major factor, and stress seems to interfere with the normal oestrogen/progesterone balance at a hypothalamus level, causing imbalance within the endometrium.

The Conventional Treatment of Dysmenorrhoea

Heat, warmth and rest are often recommended, together with a variety of analgesics of the aspirin/codeine family which may cause stomach irritation and upset. Antispasmodics such as atropine which relax smooth muscle are also commonly used. In an attempt to combat and correct the hormonal imbalance, trial and error methods are frequently used. The contraceptive pill is often given to suppress ovulation, so that progesterone build-up does not occur. Anti-prostaglandin drugs as Naprosyn or Indomethacin, which inhibit their build-up, are also tried. Various anti-inflammatory remedies are also sometimes given.

Recommended Remedies for Dysmenorrhoea

a) When the pain is predominantly before the cycle commences

1) Belladonna

There is great sensitiveness to touch and movement, so that the least jolt, perhaps in a car or train, sets off the pains, giving a low abdominal sensation of dragging weight, pulling down heavily and unpleasantly into the pelvis. The face is often typically flushed.

2) Calcarea

There is a colicky pain, often marked sweating over the whole body. There is may be a milky, thick leucorrhoeal loss which may be excoriating to the surrounding skin, which is often irritated and tender. Weakness, nausea and general illness are common.

3) Chamomilla

There is very severe colicky pain before the period, which is usually early. The whole lower abdomen and ovarian region is tender. Vomiting and sometimes diarrhoea are common. Fainting may occur with weakness. There is a characteristic violent anger, with an intolerence of any noise or interference at this time of the month, and the sufferer will need to urinate frequently.

4) Platina

There is colic, together with a cramping pain in the left ovarian region, associated with extreme vaginal hypersensitivity and constipation. Periods are early, heavy, and often dark with clots. The overall mood is one of restless agitation, suspicion and haughty authority, with underlying anxiety and an inability to relax.

b) When the pain occurs during the menstrual flow

1) China
In general the periods are both heavy and early, sometimes with the passing of dark clots in the flow. The most characteristic indications are extreme tiredness and collapse, together with low cramping colicky pains.

2) Graphites
There is severe colic, often in the lower left ovarian region, with a cycle which is often delayed and short lasting. Pruritus is common, and generalized rheumatic and chest pains may be present. The colic is of a sharp, cramping type, accompanied by nausea.

3) Nux vom.
Often the periods are early and prolonged, accompanied by cramping pains in the lower back, constipation, urinary frequency, and bladder irritation. Exhaustion and nausea are common, together with the typical nux spasms of irritability and anger.

4) Phosphorus
There are tearing contraction pains in the back, often worse at night. Anxiety, agitation and weakness are marked, the woman feels icy cold, and often has to remain in bed. Headache, palpitations and dark rings around the eyes add to a distressing and painful period, during which anguish, anxiety and fear are often marked.

5) Sepia
There are burning colicky pains in a cycle which is usually delayed and light. The pains are felt in the uterus, and are dragging and heavy, the woman often sitting tightly cross-legged as if everything would otherwise fall away from her. Exhaustion, solitary pursuits and irritability are characteristic. The pains cause restlessness and agitation. The periods are typically very irregular and unreliable, often with a dark flow, accompanied by headache, pruritus vulvae, toothache and indigestion. A burning and excoriating yellowish leucorrhoea is often present throughout the cycle.

c) When the pain is after the period

1) Lachesis
This is one of the most useful of all remedies for menstrual colicky pains. The pains are felt most of all on the left side of the abdomen and in the left ovary. The period is usually slight, often with a dark loss which may be offensive. Pains occur in the renal areas but tend to concentrate around the left ovary. Diarrhoea, a feeling as though the cervix is wide open, and intolerance of any weight or tightness around the abdominal region are characteristic.

2) Pulsatilla
One of the best remedies, indicated where the periods are very variable and changeable, and the mood is one of sadness and weeping. Usually the periods are late and slight, with colicky spasms of lower abdominal pain, nausea and diarrhoea.

3) Veratrum alb.
There is severe colic with diarrhoea and sometimes nausea and vomiting. The period is in general early and heavy, with a marked tendency to chilliness, cold sweats and pallor. Agitation, sadness and fear are often present, and are exacerbated by the period.

Amenorrhoea
Amenorrhoea is the absence of a regular menstrual cycle, where a cycle has previously been established on a normal and regular basis.

Causes of Amenorrhoea
Pregnancy is the commonest cause of absence of the menstrual cycle. Lactation also causes amenorrhoea. There is on average a twelve-week delay between delivery and the first post-partum period, and many women do not have a period at all during lactation. The first ovulation is always 'silent' and may occur at any time from the sixth week onward, and it is not at all infrequent for a woman to discover that she has become pregnant while still breast-feeding without noticing any change in her cycle at all.

Physical illness is sometimes a cause of amenorrhoea, varying from adrenal disease to thyroid disorders such as goitre or an underfunctioning of the glands. Hyperthyroidism or thyrotoxicosis with general overactivity may sometimes provoke amenorrhoea in severe cases. Diabetes is another common cause.

Stress and emotional illness are perhaps the commonest factors which inhibit ovulation and a normal cycle. Anorexia nervosa or even excessive slimming can also be a cause. Disease of the ovary, especially multiple cysts throughout the ovary (Stein-Leventhal Syndrome) may sometimes be a cause. Another rare cause, said by some authorities to account for up to ten per cent of cases, is pituitary dysfunction from the pressure of a small benign fibrous adenoma or simple fibrous tumour of the pituitary, which puts pressure on the gland and interferes with hormonal secretions.

An early menopause, occurring in the early forties, is another frequent cause. This is often hereditary. Coming off the oral contraceptive pill after many months or years of use can also cause amenorrhoea. Both the normal cycle and fertility sometimes fail to re-establish for a period of sometimes several months. Prolonged travel, especially air travel, acts as a depressant to ovulation and the normal cycle. Nightworkers often lose sense of menstrual rhythm as an occupational hazard, and women working in photographic darkrooms may also be similarly affected. Convalescence, especially from a long debilitating illness and the use of certain drugs, especially the prostaglandin inhibitors, are known in some cases to inhibit menstruation.

Symptoms of Amenorrhoea
The main symptom is the complete and total absence of the menstrual period over a period of several months, and other symptoms are rare. Pain is usually absent.

The Conventional Approaches to Amenorrhoea
This varies very much with the exact diagnosis of the problem and is treated accordingly. A physical cause such as diabetes or thyroid disease requires correction with specific remedies. An obstructive or pressure cause as with cystic disease or a pituitary adenoma requires surgical removal and correction. Where there is an obvious psychological condition, this is frequently treated by tranquillizers, anti-depressants or counselling, depending upon the facilities available and the attitudes of the individual physician. When the cause is obscure, but thought to be hormonal in origin and associated with the ovulatory cycle, then Clomiphine (Clomid) may be prescribed in an attempt to stimulate healthy ovarian functioning and re-establish ovulation.

Recommended Remedies for Amenorrhoea

1) Dulcamara
There has often been exposure to excessive cold or damp in a susceptible person. The person is often like a barometer, and can tell a change of weather that is on the way. Colds and sinusitis frequently follow a change of weather. The breasts are often painful and feel swollen and firm, tender to touch.

2) Kali. carb.
A useful and deep-acting remedy when there are the typical Kali characteristics of overweight, exhaustion, anxiety, fear, and left-sided problems and pains. Recurrent sore throats and hay fever are often present. Leucorrhoea, pruritus vulvae, and swelling of the upper eye-lids are all common.

3) Lycopodium
Vaginal dryness is almost a diagnostic indication, with burning and itching, worse after intercourse. A thick milky, excoriating leucorrhoea may be present. There may be pain of the right ovary with dragging pains. Anxiety and general nervousness are marked, with loss of confidence and weeping.

4) Pulsatilla
This remedy is one of the most valuable, and is usually prescribed at some time in the treatment. There is a combination of weakness, excessive emotion, migraines and often palpitation, diarrhoea and a variable leucorrhoea. The periods may have been suppressed by exposure to damp.

5) Silicea
Weakness and underdevelopment are indicators of this remedy, with a poor circulation and chilly extremities; even on a warm day the fingers can be 'dead' and white. Constipation is common, there is a general weakness. Depression is often marked, and the skin is frequently infected with boils or small pustules. Pruritus vulvae is frequent.

Recommended Remedies for Temporary Absence of the Period due to a Clear-cut Cause

1) Aconitum
Amenorrhoea following exposure to chill or fear.

2) Colocynth
Amenorrhoea following an explosion of uncontrollable anger.

3) Natrum mur.
Amenorrhoea following any severe emotional shock.

4) Ignatia
Where the absence follows a severe loss or grief.

5) Pulsatilla
When amenorrhoea follows exposure to damp.

Menorrhagia (Heavy Periods)

The loss during any one period can vary enormously depending on the individual. Excessive loss means an amount noticeably over and above the normal loss, usually soaking right through any tampon or pad, with the necessity to change them very frequently. Most women have a heavy flow on the first day only, but when the periods are excessive, the excessive loss can last throughout a five day period. Flooding may occur, and clotting may be a feature of the menstrual loss.

Causes of Menorrhagia

This is not an uncommon problem, especially in the forty-year-old age group. Hormonal imbalance is frequently given as the reason, with an imbalance of the oestrogen/progesterone ratios.

A variety of mechanical causes can provoke the problem, especially fibroids, a uterine tumour other than a fibroid, and a complication of an IUD contraceptive. Physical disease, especially thyroid underfunctioning or myxoedema, is often said to be associated. Obesity is certainly an associated factor of some importance. Blood diseases, including high blood-pressure and purpura, can cause an excessive tendency to bleeding. Endometriosis, especially ovarian endometriosis, where the endometrial lining layer cells have found their way into the abdominal cavity via the fallopian tubes and attached themselves to the ovary, is an increasingly important cause. Emotional tension and stress are undeniable and common causes of excessive bleeding.

The Conventional Treatment of Menorrhagia

A dilation and curettage (D & C) is one of the most commonly performed empirical treatments used by gynaecologists. When this fails, many recommend a hysterectomy when the woman no longer wishes to conceive. A more conservative approach is to use hormone replacement therapy, especially progesterone (norethisterone), and often to combine this with iron replacement for any iron-deficiency anaemia due to the abnormally heavy blood loss.

Symptoms of Menorrhagia

These may be few, but the periods are known to be heavy and often prolonged, associated with clotting in some cases and a dark, black loss. Anaemia, exhaustion, lack of energy, irritability and fatigue are all common symptoms.

Recommended Remedies for Menorrhagia

a) When the period is of normal duration

1) Belladonna

The flow is excessive and usually premature, with a mixture of clots and bright red blood. Congestion is general with the face red and the body generally feeling swollen and uncomfortable, sensitive to the very least jarring or sudden movement which exacerbates either the flow or the colicy associated pains. Headache and agitation are frequent.

2) China

In general the periods are early and very heavy, with black clots. Exhaustion and often ringing vertigo are present.

3) Crocus sat.

The discharge is heavy but usually painless. The loss is frequently dark and offensive with clot formation. Movement aggravates the loss.

4) Ipecacuanha

The loss is both forceful and bright red, the amount always excessive, often continuous. In general the period is early and there are associated sharp mid-abdominal pains which cause exhaustion and a need to lie down. Weakness and nausea, often with vomiting, are characteristic of the remedy.

5) *Nux vom.*

The periods are always unreliable and spasmodic, but usually heavy and frequently early. Colic, nausea, constipation and morning aggravation are characteristic, together with the Nux mood of irritability and anger.

6) *Sabina*

The periods are usually early and heavy, often bright red with clots. Sharp knife-like stabbing pains are often present in the uterine region or vagina, and weakness and rheumaticy pains are common. The loss tends to come in spasms and is made worse by movement or any form of heat.

b) When the period is prolonged

1) *Aconitum*

The loss is usually excessive, either bright red with clots, or a watery discharge. Agitation, red face and general congestion with collapse and weakness are common, together with anxiety, fear and fainting turns.

2) *Cuprum met.*

In general the periods are late and then prolonged, with cramping lower abdominal pains. Fear and anxiety with restlessness and aggravation by touch or cold are usual.

3) *Natrum mur.*

The periods are typically very irregular and usually heavy and prolonged. Headache and constipation are often present together with cramping lower abdominal pains and apprehension. Vaginal and general mucosal dryness is a feature, together with yawning and a tearful disposition.

4) *Secale*

There is a heavy loss of a dark liquid, often offensive and continuous. Severe menstrual cramping pains of a burning type occur in the uterus and lower abdomen. The body feels cold, but the woman herself is burning hot and cannot tolerate heat in any form. Weakness is common.

5) *Sulphur*

Useful when there is a combination of burning pains and irregular and often prolonged periods which are variable, often heavy, and usually of a thick, dark consistency with accompanying skin irritation. A thick yellowish leucorrhoeal discharge is typical, and often chronic and excoriating to the vulval skin. Use when other remedies seem well-indicated but fail to give satisfactory results.

Premenstrual Tension

Premenstrual tension is a subject that has in recent years attracted a lot of attention and publicity both from the media as well as from the professionals. The book *Once a Month* by Dr Katherina Dalton (Harvester Press, 1979) has become a classic, and is the result of many years of research and study. It is recommended as basic reading for all those who wish to be better informed about the topic, and modern advances in thinking and understanding which have taken place over the past decade. The term premenstrual tension covers the range of physical discomfort, pain and mood changes which occur in the week preceding the onset of the menstrual cycle.

Symptoms of Premenstrual Tension

By far the commonest symptoms are physical, including headache, painful breasts, water-retention amounting to as much as seven pounds weight, aching rheumaticy pains, and clumsiness. Both the common breast tenderness and the rheumatics are considered to be due to increased oestrogen levels, so that both fluid and blood circulation are increased, causing the tension symptoms and swelling of the joints. Psychological symptoms include tension, anxiety, aggression and violence, depression and lethargy. The level of circulating blood sugar is said to be lowered, together with an altered sodium/potassium balance. The onset of premenstrual tension often follows the birth of a first child, when the previous oestrogen/progesterone balance is not regained after the birth. It is usually absent in pregnancy, when in any case the normal cycles of low oestrogen and progesterone fail to occur because the foetal gonadotrophic hormones keep both, especially progesterone, to a high level.

A patient aged thirty-one, who is married with two children, described her symptoms as follows: 'I can't stand any noise or argument, especially from the children. I just get very tense with them both and scream at them as I feel so tense — it's nothing to do with them really, but I just have to let off steam in some way.' Her breasts become very tender, and one breast swells to form a lump under one armpit during this period, which has been checked and found to be normal breast tissue by her general practitioner. An odd symptom she also reports is that her teeth and gums become sensitive for ten days before her period, so that she has to use warm water on the toothbrush because cold water sets them on edge.

Another patient describes being tired and ratty for a couple of days before her period started, her eyes being particularly tired and heavy. She doesn't want to do anything, feels down in the evenings, morbid and generally depressed.

Causes of Premenstrual Tension

Most cases are considered to be progesterone deficient and high in oestrogen. Some five per cent of cases are high in blood prolactin levels, which is the pituitary hormone responsible for lactation and milk formation. Most symptoms are thought to be due to fluid retention at a brain or cerebral level.

The Conventional Treatment of Premenstrual Tension

Many treatments have been tried to counteract premenstrual tension. Among the most common are the administration of progesterone, by injection or vaginal pessary, the contraceptive pill, diuretics such as chlorthiazide, or a low salt diet. Other treatments include aspirin and various analgesics, the administration of progesterone as Norethisterone, and the prescription of tranquillizers such as Valium, vitamin B_6 (pyridoxine), sedatives, and Bromocriptine.

Recommended Remedies for Premenstrual Tension

1) Ammonium carb.

Colicky pains precede the period which is often late. The pains are frequently felt in the loin and renal areas. Toothache and dental neuralgia are a feature, together with tenderness in the upper limb and thigh areas, constipation, and a general mood of depression.

2) Belladonna

In general the remedy is indicated for severe premenstrual uterine pains and discomfort, often of a violent nature with sudden spasms of contraction, always made worse by jarring or sudden movement or pressure. Flushing heat in the face and general burning sensations are common.

3) Calcarea

The usual general sense of fatigue and weakness is increased at this time with headaches, toothache, nausea and loss of appetite. The woman is even colder than usual, with sweating in the genital area, tender or painful breasts, weak, unreliable periods, and pruritus vulvae.

4) Causticum
This remedy is associated with pains and tension coming on before the period, which is often late. The pains are colicky, and relieved by bending over. Urinary symptoms of frequency or cystitis may be present. The general mood is one of depression.

5) Kali. carb.
Renal discomfort is present, and sometimes pain, exhaustion, left-sided discomfort and anxiety, all worse in the early morning hours. There is a tendency to be accident-prone and much more tense than usual.

6) Nux vom.
Recommended when there are sudden spasms and flashes of temper or anger, often associated with an irregular cycle and pain in the first days of the flow. Constipation and urinary frequency, spasm and irritation are also common.

7) Platina
Recommended when there is pain or discomfort of a burning nature, especially in the left abdomen and left ovarian region, so that the least touch or pressure aggravates the discomfort. Libido is often heightened. The tendency to criticize others is increased, as well as feelings of jealousy and suspicion. The cycle is usually early and often painful and heavy.

8) Pulsatilla
Tears, anxiety and hysteria are all aggravated in the most variable and changeable fashion. Physical symptoms of nausea, tension, giddiness, fainting or pain are increased, and the cycle is unpredictable, changeable, and often absent or delayed and short.

9) Sepia
Exhaustion, irritability, low back pains, cramping lower abdominal tension, and colicky spasms are all common. There is almost total loss of libido, and an increase in anger and intolerance. Indifference, depression, and moodiness are all common.

Pain at Ovulation (Mittelschmerz)

This is a quite common condition associated with oestrogen build-up just prior to ovulation, when the woman experiences cramping pain and discomfort at the time of ovum release. It is basically caused by muscular spasm in the tubes and to a lesser extent in the associated ligaments, due to increased tone and the optimum positioning of the tube for ovulation. It is usually best treated symptomatically or ignored. The homoeopathic remedies are usually effective and recommended. When the pain is severe, the orthodox approach is to give either analgesic codeine-type pain killers or the oral contraceptive pill to inhibit ovulation. The latter is not recommended except in very young girls and when all other methods have failed.

Recommended Remedies for Pain at Ovulation

1) Atropine
This is a generally useful remedy for spasm in general, and often efficacious in lower abdominal and ovarian pain.

2) Colocynth
There is severe colicky and doubling-up pain often brought on by anger or irritability, or when there has been an emotional hurt.

3) Naja
Indicated when the pain or spasm affects the left ovary predominantly. Palpitations are a frequent accompanying problem, and the symptoms are usually aggravated by sleep. Depression and lack of energy are marked.

4) Nux vom.
Spasms of burning colicky pain, constipation, indigestion and flatulence, often with nausea and loss of appetite. Severe irritation and spasms of uncontrollable but short-lasting rage are common.

5) Sabina
The slightest movement or warmth serves to aggravate the ovarian discomfort. The periods are usually early, heavy, and often prolonged.

6) Staphisagria
The pains are sharp, stabbing and very severe, with considerable tenderness

to pressure or touch. The pain may radiate down to the groin or thigh regions. Indignation and anger nearly always aggravate the condition, and there is a strong sense of humiliation. Warmth gives comfort and improvement.

7) *Zincum met.*
A useful remedy where there is pain in the left ovary accompanied by nervous tension and restlessness. The spasms are helped by rest, and are often worse in the late afternoon, and worsened by pressure or touch.

Breakthrough Bleeding or Spotting
When there is an occasional vaginal loss of bright blood, not more than a few spots and always at ovulation time, this can be regarded as normal, associated with rupture of the follicle cells or a tiny blood vessel on the ovary surface. It does not necessitate any treatment. It is common at times for women on the oral contraceptive pill, is usually not exactly mid-cycle or related to ovulation, and may only occur during a few cycles in the year. If the bleeding is minimal it can be ignored, but if such bleeding is more frequent, it is probable that the woman's contraceptive pill does not suit her and should be changed. It is most common when the woman is taking the continuous progesterone pill, so that if breakthrough bleeding does become a problem she may need the combination oestrogen pill instead, or if already on one of these a pill with a higher oestrogen content. In every case such decisions are highly important and must be taken by the expert with specialized knowledge of the latest developments. Other common causes of inter-menstrual bleeding are loss from trauma of intercourse, from a cervical erosion, a polyp or cancer. Severe psychological stress is also sometimes a cause. Make sure that the blood is vaginal in origin and not from a pile, anal tear or fissure, or from a skin lesion within the vulval area.

Recommended Remedies for Breakthrough Bleeding and Spotting

1) *China*
A useful remedy for slight loss between periods, especially when there is the characteristic exhaustion, weakness and depression. Flatulence is a common problem when the remedy is indicated. The periods are usually early, and often heavy with black clots.

2) Nitric acid

When indicated there are often problems in the vulval area, especially pruritus, or cracking and soreness. The periods are nearly always early and heavy. Symptoms are often brought on by a chill or cold. The loss is generally bright red, the overall mood one of irritation and stubborn opposition.

3) Pulsatilla

Often very helpful when variability, unpredictability, and irregularity are the norm. There is always intolerance of heat, the symptoms are rarely repeated in the same way, and passive tearfulness with a tendency to hysteria characterizes the overall mood.

3.

TAMPON OR PAD

Whatever the region or organ of the body, drainage is all-important in order for healthy functioning to occur. Like the kidney, liver and intestines, the reproductive tract depends upon a flow of secretions, for blockage and stasis can quickly lead to infection, toxin-absorption and ill-health. Infection and blockage in the reproductive organs can also rapidly lead to sterility. The vagina is not just a canal for birth and the reproductive act, but the pathway of drainage for the monthly loss and its outlet, so that the uterine lining cells can be constantly renewed. The vaginal passage must be kept healthy like all the other reproductive organs, and its surface cells, like those of the uterus, are in a constant state of replacement, development and aging. The cervical mucous plug is in a similar state of flux and changing preparedness.

For all these reasons it is important to allow free drainage and simple uncomplicated absorption during a period without causing blockage, irritation or discomfort, or any condition where infection might occur or toxins be absorbed through the delicate vaginal membranes into the blood stream. Chronic irritation, toxin absorption, and blockage to the normal drainage are potentially dangerous over a long period, with a possible risk of cancer formation if neglected. These factors must be taken into account by the thinking woman when she considers her sanitary requirements to absorb the menstrual loss. The pad gives a greater degree of natural drainage and flow, whilst the tampon may offer greater absorption, be more convenient, comfortable and more easily and discretely carried and disposed of.

The choice is a personal one for each woman to make. There are few known risks from pads, but either method can cause infection when personal hygiene is neglected and faecal matter allowed to contaminate either a pad or the string of the tampon. Usually this can be easily avoided by always cleansing the anal area away from the vaginal and urethral region, and by frequent changes of pad or tampon on the heaviest days. All young girls should be taught from an early age that following a bowel motion they must cleanse themselves away from the vagina, so that this becomes a natural, instructive hygienic precaution.

Towels or pads have been used for centuries to absorb menstrual blood loss, being discarded, burned or re-laundered according to custom. Although known for many years, it is relatively recently that western women have regularly used any form of intravaginal device or tampon to absorb menstrual loss. Tampons — the word means stopper or plug — have now become widely used, overcoming fierce moral and emotional opposition. Pads had a value to the early gynaecologists because they could easily ascertain the amount and degree of menstrual loss from the number of towels used.

Some of the early devices were primitive and undesirable. A menstrual cup or 'tassette' shaped rather like an egg-cup on a short rubber stem fitted over the cervix in an attempt to catch and contain the flow. These found little favour, and although attempts have recently been made to re-introduce a similar soft-plastic device, rather than the earlier hard rubber models, there is little advantage over the original, and I doubt whether they will meet with any great enthusiasm.

The criticism of the early tampons was not entirely moral and emotional; they were also considered to be a potential source of infection and irritation. To some extent the opposition had a basis in reality, because tampons are now known to have their risks and dangers, and even the most advanced modern tampon is not without some degree of possible risk of infection. Gynaecologists are beginning to think again that the tampon may easily become an irritant and a potential block to healthy drainage, increasing the likelihood of infection.

Paradoxically it is the most modern absorbent materials which have proven to be the greatest irritants to the delicate vaginal mucosa. One model, now withdrawn, used the potentially cancer-forming absorbent polyurethane as one of its ingredients, with an emphasis on lightness and moisture-holding properties rather than health. Most of us tend to take every new design and advance as a guaranteed improvement, largely because of advanced marketing techniques which are designed to reassure and create demand, and to discourage critical thinking or objective questioning.

Pads have existed commercially since the 'twenties, replacing the squares of absorbent cloth and flannel which had previously been used and re-used for many years. In general pads are less convenient for carrying and less compact than tampons, and for a heavy period they may be less absorbent and less reliable as far as leakage is concerned. At the same time they carry far less risk of infection and irritation, or the toxic reabsorption side effect.

Tampons were first marketed commercially in 1936. Tampax was the first model to be readily available, and was designed by a doctor. Various other internal absorbent materials had been used for many years by women before the cotton tampax came into general use. Some of the early materials were of vegetable fibre origin; papyrus for example was used by Egyptian women. Wool inserts were popular with the Romans, whilst the Japanese used a form of absorbent paper. South Pacific women preferred a soft grass material to absorb the monthly loss, and other cultures have used sea sponge for many generations. Attempts have been made in recent years to make these sponges acceptable alternatives to the modern tampon, but unfortunately they are often contaminated because of widespread sea pollution, and are not often recommended because of the dangers of infection.

Over the years, tampons have given rise to contradictory and varied opinions as to their potential danger from irritation, infection and re-absorption. According to some sources, tampons increase cramps and period pains because of a suction-like effect upon the uterus. There is little doubt that a tampon may cause considerable pain and discomfort from pressure upon a sensitive cervix or on the pelvic ligaments. In general it is best to use a tampon which stretches and absorbs the menstrual fluid by swelling and expanding widthways rather than in length, so that there is minimum risk of pressure on the cervix.

Tampons should never be used between periods to absorb or eliminate normal discharge and moisture. Many cases of vaginal irritation, ulceration and infection have now been definitely associated with tampons. In recent years, but particularly since 1978, toxic shock syndrome (TSS) has become increasingly recognized and reported as a complication of tampon usage. Most common in young women from fifteen to twenty-five, severe symptoms usually occur on the third or fourth day of the period, with a raised temperature, nausea, vomiting and shock. Diarrhoea may occur and headache is common, with a typical and diagnostic peeling rash which resembles sun-burn and occurs mainly on the hands and feet. Sore throat, conjunctivitis, and in severe cases a lowered blood-pressure occur, with kidney or liver failure and cardiac weakness, sometimes with aneurysm formation. The cause of TSS is thought to be a very severe reaction to toxin infection by the dangerous staphylococcus aureus. All reported cases have occurred in women, at the time of their period, who had been using tampons. Many were using a particular brand which has now been withdrawn from the market, and usually of the super-absorbent kind. Tampons may damage the vaginal wall, causing pain when they are removed, and creating a potential pathway for toxin reabsorption and infection. To be on the safe side, always use a tampon with care and thoughtful caution. Change them frequently, avoid their use when the flow is minimal, being especially cautious of the super-absorbent type.

The other common problem associated with tampons is recurrent vaginal yeast infection or trichomonas. Ulceration is also frequent, both of the cervix and vaginal wall, the reason not always being completely understood. Menstrual cramp is a very common problem, and some gynaecologists believe that tampon usage may cause a blockage and reversal of the normal direction of menstrual flow so that loss occurs via the fallopian tubes and endometrial cells and tissues, causing endometriosis. This has become an increasingly common condition in recent years, with a 'seeding' of menstrual cells into the abdominal peritoneal cavity, especially around the ovaries and uterus, but also around other inner abdominal organs, being responsible for many cases of menstrual pain and cramp.

Minor itchy irritation and eczema may also occur, sometimes of an allergic nature, and dryness may be a complication. Slight haemorrhage is not uncommon, especially when plastic inserters have been used. Rash in the vulval region may be a complication of tampon usage, also sometimes causing recurrent cystitis and 'spotting' between periods. In some cases the menstrual cycles may also become more prolonged. The string is always a potential source of infection from anal contamination, and is an important reason why the tampon must be changed frequently.

Tampons have not been sterilized since the early days, when ethylene oxide gas was used. This is now, however, considered to be toxic, and only a few countries still use the original method. In general, both tampons and pads are sold unsterilized. The deodorant tampon is definitely not recommended, and many have now been withdrawn from the market, because of the risks of allergic reaction. In general avoid any tampon that is either dry or uncomfortable, which 'pulls' or is difficult to remove. When using them it should not be forgotten that any tampon may be a potential source of infection and irritation, that it is a foreign body, that it may be potentially dangerous to your health and well-being, and that however efficient its absorbent properties, tampons should always be treated with thoughtful care.

Many women could benefit from a rest period away from the constant prolonged use of tampons from time to time, perhaps for two to three cycles in a year. During this time the use of pads encourages freer drainage. When this has been carried out, many women have found that certain irritations and vulval rashes clear up, even when they were not obviously associated with tampon use. Few women want to go back completely to the pad after the convenience of tampons, and would regard the suggestion as an impossible one. If, however, you are getting symptoms of irritation or discomfort, do consider a break from the tampon for one or two cycles to see if there is any improvement without them. Avoid the super-absorbent types unless your period is very heavy, and on heavy days consider using a pad. The use of more than one intra-vaginal tampon has nothing to recommend it, and the practice should be avoided.

There are no specific recommendations for homoeopathic treatments in this area, and treatment should be according to symptoms. In general there is a good response to homoeopathy provided that when the cause of a problem is from irritation the irritant is immediately removed. Toxic shock syndrome, with collapse, low blood pressure and cardiac weakness, vomiting and shock, requires urgent and immediate hospitalization, often with fluid intravenous replacement. Homoeopathy should not be attempted in such circumstances, and the care of the patient must be in medical hands.

4.

PREGNANCY

Morning Sickness

Morning sickness, as nausea of pregnancy is usually called, is something of a misnomer. It is especially common in the morning hours, but may occur throughout the day, and during the whole of the pregnancy. It occurs in 50-60 per cent of pregnancies, and although the exact cause is unknown, it is usually considered to be a gastrointestinal response to the hormonal changes of pregnancy, and particularly to oestrogen levels. The onset is usually early, in the fifth week, frequently lasting into the twelfth week. Sometimes it occurs almost immediately after conception, so that it is the very earliest sign of pregnancy, even before a period is missed.

Causes of Morning Sickness

Morning sickness is the result of hormonal imbalance, especially high oestrogen levels acting via the hypothalamus upon the gastrointestinal organs. The major hormonal change that takes place during early pregnancy is the outpouring of chorionic gonadotrophins (within a few hours of conception occurring) by the dividing cells of the fertilized ovrum as it passes along the fallopian tube, which prevents menstruation destroying the early embedding process. The gonadotrophins prevent the levels of progesterone, and to a lesser extent oestrogen, from dropping. The corpus luteum is the early source of this hormone output but soon the young placenta takes over to produce enough oestrogen and progesterone for a healthy pregnancy. This developing corpus luteum is vital in these first twelve weeks of pregnancy, and during this time it may become enlarged or cystic, and often tender because of its degree of activity. Tender, painful intercourse may be a symptom of the extremely sensitive ovarian corpus during this stage of overactivity.

Symptoms of Morning Sickness
The main symptoms are nausea, vomiting and loss of appetite. The least smell of food brings on nausea and sickness, which if continuous and severe may cause weight loss, dehydration and even jaundice. When this occurs hospitalization may be required and intravenous fluid replacement necessary to preserve the health of the foetus and mother.

The Conventional Approach to Morning Sickness
For many years treatment was conservative and careful, but in the 1960s Distabal (Thalidomide) was often a recommended 'effective' treatment of morning sickness, and was considered a breakthrough cure until the side-effects upon the foetus were revealed. Present day attitudes are fortunately much more cautious because foetal risks are better understood. Bicarbonate of soda is often recommended as an antacid. The frequent eating of dry biscuits or toast and an apple is well-supported and recommended. Vitamins, especially B_6, are said to be helpful and effective in some cases. Iron is often prescribed.

Recommended Remedies for Morning Sickness

1) Antimonium Tartrate
Useful when vomiting occurs immediately after having eaten, usually of undigested food, and typically accompanied by collapse and exhaustion. A lot of mucus is produced and present in the vomit, which is thick and often white or mixed with bile. The mucus is sometimes stringy. Vomiting is usually spasmodic, sudden and severe.

2) Argentum Nitricum
Indicated when there is very considerable flatulence accompanying the nausea and vomiting. There is frequently a craving for sugar and sweet foods, and panicy nervousness is characteristic. All forms of heat are abhorrent, and cool fresh air is sought.

3) Ipecacuanha
One of the best remedies for constant and persistent nausea and vomiting with excessive salivation. Mucus and bile are often present in the vomit.

Thirst is noticeably absent, and there is irritability of mood.

4) Nux vom.
Indicated when vomiting occurs in sudden spasms after breakfast, with a bitter acid-tasting vomit. The lower stomach feels as though it contains a heavy weight, and constipation with very marked irritability completes the indications.

5) Petroleum
In spite of the persistent nausea and vomiting, the woman never loses her appetite, and after vomiting returns immediately to eating.

6) Pulsatilla
Variable nausea, with an intolerance of heat, or of anything greasy or fatty. The symptoms often come on in the afternoon or evening, but are typically changeable. There is an absence of thirst, and in general only cold acidic drinks are acceptable. There is often a thick whitish-yellow coating to the tongue, and the general mood is one of tearful passivity.

7) Sepia
In spite of the symptoms there is no lack of appetite, and hunger is often seemingly insatiable. The vomit is often pale with mucus, and is followed by exhaustion and fatigue, constipation and irritability. Low dragging abdominal pains with a general sensation of emptiness is characteristic. Indifference is often diagnostic.

8) Sulphur
There is a burning acid vomit with an offensive odour. Hunger is marked, and often the vomiting or a sense of weight-like discomfort occurs soon after eating. Symptoms are often worse on waking. Diarrhoea is common, as is some form of skin itching.

9) Tabacum
Useful when there is nausea, pallor, chilliness and persistent salivation.

Recurrent Miscarriage
Although the statistics are often misleading, about 15 to 20 per cent of all pregnancies are said to end in spontaneous miscarriage or abortion. The loss of a pregnancy, unless it occurs very early and is almost unnoticed is,

in the majority of cases, profoundly upsetting psychologically and emotionally. Where miscarriage is deliberately induced a different set of emotions may occur, but they are just as disturbing. In its early weeks, when the embedding process is taking place, the young embryo is particularly vulnerable to abortion. It may occur at any time, but is especially frequent in the third month, from the eleventh week onwards. The twelfth and fourteenth weeks are particular danger times, with an additional time of vulnerability in some cases from the sixth week onwards. The condition is often recurrent.

Symptoms of Recurrent Miscarriage
The recurrence of intra-uterine foetal loss associated with a vaginal discharge of blood and accompanying cramping abdominal pains of uterine origin.

Causes of Recurrent Miscarriage
All too often the causes are not known, and miscarriage is a sudden crisis in an otherwise normal and desired pregnancy, free from any obvious underlying psychological stresses or precipitating causes. The major cause is thought to be hormonal failure at the time when progesterone production from the corpus luteum is reduced and the young placenta is taking over its production. At this time progesterone output may be incomplete, so that spontaneous abortion easily occurs without warning, the chorionic foetal gonadotrophins being insufficient to maintain the required basic progesterone levels.

In about half of cases the cause is thought to be a genetic abnormality of the foetus leading to abnormal development and implantation. Disease and ill-health of the mother are also important, especially such chronic problems as diabetes, kidney infections like nephritis, and german measles. Thyroid disorder and infections can lower maternal health and endanger the young foetus. Hypertension or raised blood-pressure is another important cause of maternal ill-health and foetal loss.

Any anomaly or abnormality of the uterus can be a cause of miscarriage, including fibroids, cervical weakness and the fusion of one area of the uterus. Malpositioning can be a contributory factor, as in retroversion, when the uterus is tipped backwards. This may cause the foetus to fail to embed itself, or to grow with the speed and within the space required. In recent years it has become apparent that hereditary influences are a major factor in miscarriage, accounting for as much as 50 per cent of cases. Fortunately these reasons are mostly non-recurrent, so that a subsequent pregnancy has a good chance of being unaffected.

Hormonal causes have been already mentioned, and an underfunctioning thyroid gland can play a decisive role in miscarriage, because metabolism and the other processes of development and functioning tend to be slowed down and interfered with, including the vital embedding process. Sexual intercourse can provoke a miscarriage, but in most cases there is probably already a pre-existing abnormality. Accidental injury, shock and accidents are much more common causes of miscarriage. Certain drugs such as lead, quinine and colchicine — a remedy for gout — are dangerous in pregnancy. High levels of lead in the environment are a danger to foetal development, and this may stimulate more effective legislation and safeguards than at present are provided for.

Causes connected with the paternal sperm are not yet fully understood, but the connection is probably chromosomal, where there is incompatibility with the partner. If a child is conceived with another partner there may be no recurrence of the miscarriages. The final and sometimes most important factor is psychological; shock, fear, loss or anxiety act powerfully on the hypothalamus, and can easily upset the closely related pituitary output and control mechanisms.

The Conventional Approach to Recurrent Miscarriage

Treatment is still not very satisfactory in many cases and is often empirical. For many, the best treatment is prevention during a subsequent pregnancy. Rest and quiet are essential in all cases, with a minimum of disturbance and avoidance of coitus. Some surgeons have tried to put a stitch in the os cervix for a threatened mid-term miscarriage and, with bed rest, results are encouraging, but this treatment does little to prevent the early inevitable cases. Other doctors recommend folic acid supplements or implants in an attempt to reduce haemorrhage and developmental abnormalities. The B_6 hormone may also be given by injection, but this carries the very real risk of virilizing or masculinizing the foetus, which is particularly undesirable with a female foetus. Sometimes there is a slight brownish discharge which occurs in the early weeks, but without pain. With quiet and rest this often passes without further problems. This sort of discharge is not the inevitable abortion which follows severe cramping pains and a brown or bright red haemorrhagic loss.

Whenever a miscarriage is in any way incomplete — either from a retained placenta or retention of foetal remnants, a D&C is recommended. This surgical scraping-out and cleansing of the uterus is absolutely essential in all cases, and if neglected there can be a real danger to the mother of infection or interference with subsequent pregnancies. Some gynaecologists use pure progesterone suppositories or pessaries.

Recommended Remedies for Recurrent Miscarriage

a) Where there is a history of recurrent miscarriage

1) *Calcarea*
When there is a light and pale haemorrhagic loss, often from an apparently trivial emotional problem in a woman of obese disposition who is too easily tired and often chilly.

2) *Carbo veg.*
There is just a slight loss of bright red blood as a warning of a recurrent problem. Flatulence and chilliness are marked.

3) *Ferrum met.*
Recommended for the woman who is anaemic but easily flushed. Exhaustion is typical, sometimes with shortness of breath. When bleeding occurs it is usually slight and pale.

4) *Pulsatilla*
This is recommended when there are irregular pains or a slight loss, the condition is variable and the woman is chilly but intolerant of heat. Tears, absence of thirst, diarrhoea, and a quiet passive temperament are most indicative.

5) *Sabina*
This remedy helps to prevent as well as treat recurrent miscarriage around the twelfth week. The main symptoms are pain in the renal area and down the abdomen into the thigh area. There is great sensitivity to heat, as well as an intolerance of jarring or movement. The woman is often overweight, with a history of heavy, prolonged periods.

6) *Sepia*
One of the major and most useful remedies after pulsatilla and sabina. The indications are dragging, weight-like pains in the lower back and abdomen, accompanied by exhaustion, indifference, irritability, hunger, constipation, a yellowish skin discolouration, and late light periods. Toothache and

migrainous headaches are both frequent before periods, and may occur during the pregnancy.

b) Where there is a threat to an existing pregnancy
Remember: the treatment of a threatened abortion should always be by a doctor.

1) Arnica
Often the first remedy to give, especially where there has been any shock or profuse loss of blood.

2) Belladonna
One of the major remedies for the condition. There are often violent uterine contractions and a loss of bright blood, the uterus and vaginal area being very tender to the least touch or pressure. An overpowering tiredness is characteristic, as is hypersensitivity to noise, smells, pressure or movement. Low sacral back pain is severe, and there is a general sense of downward pressure.

3) Sabina
Painful uterine contractions are indicative, followed by the expulsion of dark clots and a bright red loss. Itching and shooting pains from the sacrum towards the vagina are characteristic, as well as an intolerance of heat and a craving for fresh air.

4) Secale
There is a discharge of dark offensive black blood in a woman who is often thin and pale, exhausted and weak with little reserve of energy. Diarrhoea is common.

5.

BREAST-FEEDING PROBLEMS

Breast development is one of the first external signs of puberty or sexual maturing, and begins two or three years before the onset of menstruation. These early signs may begin from the age of seven or eight depending upon the individual girl and her inherited characteristics. The protruding nipple, surrounded by a pink areola which slowly darkens with maturity, is pushed outwards by growth of the underlying glandular tissue of breast buds. Sometimes one breast may at times be larger than the other, and they may occasionally be painful as blood levels of oestrogens rise and fall in early puberty. The quiescent milk ducts develop from the age of fifteen or sixteen, and are enveloped in fat, separated into some fifteen to twenty-five lobules, each with its alveoli, creating a branched and tree-like system of milk-producing cells and their ducts.

Lactation
Milk production begins just before childbirth, as oestrogen and progesterone levels fall. The hypothalamus is triggered to inform the anterior pituitary to produce the hormone prolactin, which is the stimulus to milk production. With a first baby, the initial secretion is the highly nutritious thick yellow-coloured fluid called colostrum. It is present from the last few weeks of pregnancy, and is important because it contains protective antibodies. The young baby takes in the colostrum when first put to the breast, receiving maternal antibodies at an early stage. Breast milk is formed and present from the third day with a first baby, although often sooner with a second and subsequent pregnancies. The sucking reflex of the child at the nipple stimulates a nervous pathway to the hypothalamus so that the other major

hormone concerned in milk release, oxytocin, is produced by the pituitary gland. This causes the 'letting down' or contraction of the alveoli, and the flow of milk from the glandular alveoli to the nipple. Usually the forceful flow of milk starts about twenty seconds from the moment of the first sucking, which stimulates the reflex action to commence.

During pregnancy the breasts naturally enlarge and are often heavy, but breast size is no indication of milk production and quality. It is often a smaller breast which produces better quality of milk than heavier larger breasts, although there are exceptions to this. A smaller breast has the advantage of less fatty tissue and a greater development of active glandular elements. It is the latter which are responsible for the amount and quality of the milk, rather than the enveloping fat which is largely protective in function.

Normal Cyclical Breast Changes

Changes occur each month not only in the uterine lining cells, but also in the alveolar cells of the breasts. The stimulation and growth of the breast is governed by the same hormonal output as the endometrium, the vaginal mucosa, the cervix and the fallopian tubes. The breasts share in these cyclical changes, which are a preparation for the possibility of pregnancy. Such breast changes vary in degree and discomfort with the individual woman.

During the early part of the menstrual cycle, the cycle is dominated by oestrogen release, which stimulates the lactation ducts into a new and renewed phase of growth, proliferation and development. In the later stage of the cycle, progesterone release from the corpus luteum causes this growth and activity to reach a maximum in the duct cells as well as in the alveoli, which tend to swell. As in the uterus at this time in the cycle, there is a very considerable increase in blood flow and fluid content, so there is often an increased awareness of the breasts being firmer and heavier. In a sensitive woman breast discomfort and pain may occur. Where a woman is taking a combination of oestrogen contraceptive pill to suppress ovulation, the breast discomfort may be increased. Never take the pill during lactation, as it is a dangerous risk to the baby's health.

Fertility During Lactation

There is a common fallacy that a lactating woman cannot conceive, and this has been quite commonly used as a totally unreliable means of contraception by many women. Although it is usual not to menstruate during this period, fertility and ovulation usually continues. Many women are fertile shortly after the baby is born, so from the earliest days contraceptive precautions must be taken, and these should preferably be of a mechanical kind for the duration of lactation.

Painful Breasts during Breast-feeding

Pain in the breasts is usually due to hardness or tenderness, either from the increase in milk production, or with a baby who for a variety of reasons is not sucking well or strongly enough for the amount of milk produced. When there is an excess of milk formed, for whatever reason, it is best removed manually by means of a breast pump. Sometimes when the nipples are small and the breast tense, the baby just cannot obtain an adequate sucking grip on the breast to suck properly, and the breasts can become painful. Suppression of lactation may be necessary if the pain is severe.

The Conventional Approach to Painful Breast Problems

Approaches to this problem vary considerably. Diuretics are sometimes used to try and reduce the amount of fluid retention and vascularization of the breast. Bandaging the breasts tightly is a classic and frequent recipe for the condition, which may give some relief. Purgatives have been tried in the past in order to eliminate body fluids generally and relieve the pressure and tension in the breasts. For similar reasons keeping fluid intake to a minimum may be recommended, in order to reduce milk production. Hormonal treatments are also used in some cases, but they are in general unwise and a potential hazard to the baby. Oxytocin as a nasal spray may be prescribed to stimulate the ducts.

Recommended Remedies for Painful Breasts

1) Bryonia

Certainly one of the best and most useful remedies, where there is a firm or hard discomfort. The breast is often hot, but the overlying skin is of normal colour. It is reputed to have most effect when the left breast is affected, but it is always a basic remedy to use.

2) Belladonna

This remedy follows Bryonia closely in value. The breasts are hard with sometimes tearing pains, but there is much more heat and redness of the overlying skin. The mother is often restless, and the breasts are extremely sensitive to touch or movement.

3) Calcarea
This may help where the problem is more right-sided, the breast tense and painful, but without heat, generally pale, and damp from perspiration.

4) Phellandrium
This is useful if the pains tend to occur mainly when the infant is suckling.

5) Phytolacca
Indicated for severe hardness and induration of the breast, especially for a painful and tender left breast.

6) Aconitum
Indicated for the sudden onset of painful breasts. Use this remedy only during the early stages, and preferably during the first forty-eight hours of the problem.

7) Mercurius
Indicated when the pain is due to an infection or a threatened abscess. The breast is hard and tender, and the temperature may be elevated.

Excess Milk During Lactation
This is not uncommon, and occurs when lactation is produced in excess of the infant's needs. It is sometimes a problem when there have been several previous pregnancies, and breast development and glandular output has increased with each successive pregnancy. The breast is painful or uncomfortable, the milk leaks from the nipple, and the mother may become very uncomfortable and constantly damp around the breast from loss of milk. The breast becomes hard from too much milk production and insufficient sucking and demand by the infant.

The Conventional Approach to Excess Milk During Lactation
The commonest approach is the extraction of any excess milk with a breast pump. The milk can be stored and used for supplementary feeding or for other infants. Binders have been used for this problem for many years, usually as tight bandaging of the breast area in an attempt to reduce glandular output and to provide support to relieve discomfort and pain. Hormones are sometimes recommended, but they are most definitely not advised as a safe treatment.

Recommended Remedies for Excess Milk During Lactation

1) Borax
Milk overflows freely between feeds, and the milk is often thick. An odd but important characteristic symptom is pain or discomfort in the opposite breast to the one where the infant is sucking. Anxiety and fear is marked, the nervousness aggravated by downward movements such as walking downstairs or leaning forwards.

2) Calc. carb.
Indicated for a pale, tired, overweight woman, who is often covered with sweat.

3) China
This is indicated where there is excess milk production associated with the most extreme weakness and debility.

4) Natrum mur.
Recommended when there is a combination of obesity and congestion, especially of the chest region and the breasts, which are hypersensitive and tender to the least pressure. There is a generally poor state of health, and damp in any form aggravates the condition.

5) Phosphorus
There is an excess flow often associated with feelings of heaviness and heat in the opposite breast.

6) Pulsatilla
Usually the best remedy in a chilly, emotional and passive disposition. The flow is variable, sometimes excessive but at other times the feed is normal. Heat in any form aggravates the condition.

7) Rhus tox.
Recommended when there is a general tenderness and overall distention of the breasts with tenderness and an itching discomfort.

Insufficient Milk Production
There is not enough milk produced by the glandular tissue of the breasts for the needs of the baby. The causes are not always clear. The sucking

reflex is the best stimulus for milk production, and when it is weak there may not be sufficient stimulus of the hypothalamus to produce oxytocin and contraction of the milk ducts. In some cases the baby is weak or premature, in others the mother is ill or suffering from psychological shock, illness, trauma or grief. In most cases, however, the cause is not so clearly marked. At present the artificial and chemical stimulus of milk from the breast is unsatisfactory and not recommended. In all cases, excessive painful sucking over a prolonged period should be avoided because of the risks of damage to the nipple, infection, and possible abscess formation in severe cases. The infant may lose weight because of insufficient nutritional intake, and may need supplements in one form or other.

The Conventional Approach to Insufficient Milk Production
The usual approach is to continue breast-feeding as long as possible, so that the infant can take in whatever breast milk is being formed. In this way the baby is felt to be receiving both physical and psychological gains. Food supplements of cow's milk and solids are also be given, depending upon the age and weight of the baby.

Recommended Remedies for Insufficient Milk Production

1) Agnus cast.
The milk flow ceases soon after onset or quickly becomes reduced. The general picture is of maternal weakness with pallor and anaemia.

2) Asafoetida
After about the tenth day, the milk supply reduces and dries up. There is an overall general problem of maternal flatulence, an offensive catarrh, and often a sense of generalized numbness.

3) Causticum
From the start the flow is weak. Other indicators are anxiety, fatigue and insomnia.

4) Pulsatilla
The best remedy after Agnus cast., indicated by a weak flow which is typically variable and changeable.

5) *Urtica Urens*
For use where there is a total absence of milk associated with stinging, itching irritating discomfort, and pains in the breast areas and often elsewhere.

Recommended Remedies when the Milk has been Suddenly Suppressed due to a Clear-cut Event

1) *Dulcamara* or *Pulsatilla*
Where there has been exposure to sudden cold and chill or damp.

2) *Ignatia* or *Phosphoric acid*
When there is sudden and acute grief or psychological shock.

3) *Natrum mur.*
Where there is a sudden suppression of lactation following an acute emotional experience.

4) *Chamomilla*
When there has been loss of control after a severe outburst of anger.

5) *Aconitum*
Where acute fear has caused the suppression.

Painful Nipples
The nipples and areola need careful looking after during pregnancy to prevent cracking and infection. Firming, drawing-out, gentle rolling and towel massage is recommended. Lanolin may be used to toughen the nipple and to avoid cuts and sores. The regular use of calendula cream is the homoeopathic alternative to lanolin. During feeding the infant may fail to grip the whole of the areola if the nipple is not inserted correctly. In such cases the baby may manipulate the firm but vulnerable nipple, causing cracking. There is a technique to breast-feeding which is usually learned quite spontaneously, but sometimes help is required to prevent soreness and infection from occurring.

The Conventional Approach to Painful Nipples
Antiseptic creams are often used and applied locally to the sore area. A nipple shield may be used. Where there is an excess of milk, a breast pump can be used to prevent overengorgement and soreness. Stopping feeding on the

side of the painful nipple, or use a breast shield, for a short period is sometimes recommended until the crack or condition has healed. The cause is often considered to be a staphylococcal bacterial invasion of the area. Many gynaecologists consider that prevention is generally the best treatment. Others recommend Bromocriptine in controlled usage.

Recommended Remedies for Painful Nipples

1) Arnica
May be used to prevent the condition occurring in women with a previous history of the condition when breast-feeding. Use in the sixth potency from the start of lactation.

2) Calendula.
May be applied very effectively to treat the problem locally, but it is also helpful when taken internally in the sixth potency.

3) Castor equi.
Often a very useful remedy, but use it only if graphites is insufficient.

4) Graphites
The best and most useful remedy for women with a problem of fissure or cracked, cut and sore nipples during breast-feeding.

5) Chamomilla
Useful for painful nipple conditions without the obvious cracks and sores of graphites. Breast-feeding is often associated with sharp cramping pains in the lower back, sacral region or lower abdomen each time the breast is given.

6) Nitric acid
Often used when the prevalent symptom is of splinter-like pain, the nipple tender, cracked and split.

7) Nux vom.
The nipple is painful, severely chapped and sore around the areola region. Constipation, flatulence, indigestion and irritability are marked.

8) Silicea
A general remedy to be considered for a combination of sore, cracked or

infected nipples, and weakness and a chilly disposition. A purulent discharge from the infected area of skin is characteristic.

9) Sulphur
One of the best remedies where there is soreness, chapping or redness without cracking or fissure formation. The area is very tender, and there is frequently a local skin eruption. Diarrhoea is common, especially on waking. Use this remedy early if a burning discomfort develops.

Breast Abscess
Fortunately this has now become a rather rare condition, although it was very common in the past and caused severe problems for many mothers. Nevertheless it is still the commonest breast infection in breast-feeding women. It often follows a sore or cracked nipple condition. In general the breast is painful, often red and pulsating, and at times stony hard. A high temperature is nearly always present, unless the condition has become chronic as with a cold abscess. When the condition is severe it can cause a generalized toxaemia and in one case, reported recently by a colleague, the toxic reaction provoked an acute psychotic breakdown.

The Conventional Approach to Breast Abscess
Antibiotics are the usual approach, and high levels of penicillin or tetracycline are frequently given. Incision and surgical drainage may be indicated where there is severe pus formation under pressure.

Recommended Remedies for Breast Abscess
This condition must be always under medical care. If a severe or toxic reaction sets in, with no response to homoeopathy, the patient should be under expert care and a course of antibiotics administered immediately.

1) Bryonia
The most important early remedy. The breast is inflamed and stony-hard, sensitive to touch and movement, with a sense of heaviness. Give this remedy early when an abscess is threatened.

2) Belladonna
The best remedy to follow bryonia when an abscess is beginning to form, with characteristic tenderness, heat, and redness of the overlying breast.

3) Calendula
May be applied locally as a cream or tincture to give some comfort and relief.

4) Hepar sulph.
Useful when there is local pain and soreness from infection, together with marked irritability. Where there is a marked infection it follows Mercurius in importance of depth and speed of action.

5) Merc. sol.
Usually indicated when Belladonna fails to control the situation. There is a much more toxic inflammatory reaction with profuse sweating of the whole body, raised temperature and exhaustion.

6) Phytolacca
The breast is hard and tender, and there is a combination of backache, shivering, and a raised temperature.

7) Silicea
There is an abscess which is producing a purulent discharge. The nipple area is often cracked and infected. Weakness, chilliness and exhaustion are marked.

Aversion to Breast-feeding
Although for most women breast-feeding is a most desirable and natural activity, and a disappointment when it cannot be experienced, for some women the whole idea of breast-feeding is distasteful. The feelings are of course personal and individual, and part of a complex psychological state. There may have been prolonged vomiting throughout pregnancy and a state of unrecognized or more obvious depression after the birth. Harmony in the marital relationship may leave much to be desired, the mother may have been abandoned by the father, the pregnancy unwanted or only accepted with marked ambivalent feelings. For some mothers the whole idea of physical contact with body discharges, including changing nappies and attending to vomit and breast milk, has become associated with distaste and something not nice or natural.

Although most people recommend breast-feeding as the ideal for both mother and child, it must feel right for the individual woman concerned whatever others do or recommend. The ultimate choice is the mother's, and her attitudes towards mothering her baby are what matters most — not what others say or recommend.

The Conventional Approach to Aversion to Breast-feeding

In a modern clinic, counselling is usually available, although it may be brief, and there is usually no intention to embark on a long period of prolonged therapy. Unfortunately psychological counselling is still a luxury in many maternity and neonatal units, and this is regrettable. Wherever there is a high level of caring for both mother and infant psychological consultation and counselling should be readily available.

Recommended Remedy for Aversion to Breast-feeding

Sepia

Undoubtedly this is the most consistently reliable remedy for the problem, which in most cases is best combined with counselling. Use Sepia in the sixth potency, three times daily.

6.

PUERPERAL PROBLEMS

A psychologically well-prepared and accepted pregnancy is usually a cause for joy, and ambivalent feelings are minimal. An open sharing of the coming event, both between the couple and more widely within the circle of friends and family, is one of the best natural remedies for the prevention of puerperal 'blues'. Where there is an unwanted pregnancy with a definite risk of puerperal illness, depression, or any threat to the health of the mother, the pregnancy can usually be legally terminated at an early stage with a minimum of fuss. If you come into this category and are depressed and pregnant, then get help as early as possible in the pregnancy to prevent technical problems interfering with a late termination. If you are in doubt, then discuss the problem with your own doctor, or telephone an organization like the Samaritans for advice.

When there is such a problem during a pregnancy, then specialized pregnancy counselling is usually available. The physician-in-charge should also be able to help with any doubts or feelings which seem unnatural and difficult to live with. If you have a good relationship with your family doctor, then chat to him, in order to try and put any distortions, doubts and fears back into perspective, and pave the way for an uneventful, smooth after-birth period.

The period of birth and confinement has changed appreciably for the better over recent years in the majority of clinics and obstetric units. The presence and active support of the husband during the birth has been of enormous emotional consequence to both partners. It provides support for the mother, and helps the father to feel much more involved, but most importantly, it paves the way for psychologically healthy puerperal time.

The time following the birth is a very vulnerable time for every woman.

The predominant needs are for closeness, understanding and sensitivity because of the psychological, hormonal, physiological and sociological pressures and changes. It is important that confidence and sharing be at a maximum during this period to avoid any sense of 'let down' when the pregnancy is finally over.

Puerperal Depression

This is an extremely common but usually misunderstood condition. Feeling low and down-spirited can easily become a source of anxiety and guilt to the mother, because she feels that she has everything to be happy for and ought not to be feeling anything other than fully contented and satisfied. A temporary psychological 'low' is common to most mothers on about the third day after the birth, which often coincides with the establishment of breast feeding.

Some women do not seem to recover from this depression, and go on to become increasingly depressed, tired, irritable and often exhausted. The low-spirited mood may improve quite spontaneously, but sometimes frightening and ambivalent feelings start to creep in — towards the baby, breast feeding, the husband or the family. If this becomes a severe preoccupation it may lead to severe depression and sometimes to thoughts of suicide. In a severe state an acute psychotic illness can occur with hallucinations, delusions, suspicion, jealousy, and often violent fantasies. There is a sense of failure and of letting the family down. Disinterest and indifference to others is sometimes a feature, and there may be a total loss of any sexual interest.

The Conventional Approach to Puerperal Depression

The usual approach is psychological treatment either by a general physician or a psychiatrist, often combined with the use of anti-depressants and tranquillizers.

Recommended Remedies for Puerperal Depression

1) Aconitum

I prefer to use this remedy for an acute state of depression rather than for a chronic problem. The exception to this is an emotional depressive state which has been brought on by a sudden shock. The main indications are a combination of fear and agitation, often the conviction of imminent death. Congestion is general and the face may be markedly flushed. The person is usually well-built. Agitation and restlessness are also characteristic.

2) Aurum met.

This is best indicated for a combination of hopeless despair, sadness and a determined intention towards suicide. Usually there are characteristic accompanying cardiac symptoms — palpitations, chest pains, or raised blood-pressure.

3) Belladonna

This is often a useful remedy where there is a combination of restlessness, depression, a high temperature, and red, flushed features.

4) Hyoscyamus

A remedy that has been used successfully for this condition for many years. There is usually a combination of jealousy, restless agitation and depression.

5) Ignatia

Useful when the depression has been precipitated by an acute loss of any kind, the mother usually weeping silently, withdrawn and distressed.

6) Pulsatilla

This remedy is very useful in mild post-puerperal depressive states. There is mixed hysteria and sadness, with a changeable and unpredictable mood. The mother is usually very tearful and intolerant of the least heat. Thirst is absent.

7) Natrum mur.

This remedy is indicated for cases which are slightly more severe than those where Pulsatilla is indicated. The typical picture is of sadness with irritability, an inability to concentrate, and a desire to be left alone. This latter symptom contrasts it with Pulsatilla, where the mother usually wants to be in the company of others.

8) Sepia

The most useful of all remedies and the first one to be considered. The picture is typically one of weakness, sadness and tiredness. A sense of indifference to everything and everybody is marked, together with obstinate constipation, constant hunger and a yellowish-brown facial discolouration.

9) Stramonium

I recommend this remedy only if the depression involves delusions and is destructive and violent. The patient cannot rest, disturbs everyone around her with her restless agitation and insomnia. A high temperature and a red face are common.

Obesity Following Childbirth

The cause is usually psychological, although hormonal imbalance must also be considered. Mothers usually come for treatment six months to a year after birth, and often there has been a period of depression or anxiety following the birth. One mother discovered that her young baby was not moving one limb freely after the baby returned home with her from hospital. The baby was eventually discovered to have a fracture of the femur since birth, which had not been diagnosed. The child needed to be readmitted for surgical alignment and plastering of the leg. The child was a first baby, only conceived after a very lengthy period of infertility, and remained in hospital for six weeks. During this period the woman's fears and anxiety increased, even though the child made steady and good progress. The mother compensated for these pressures by a marked gain in weight because of lack of exercise and constant snack meals between visits to the clinic. Attempts to diet and exercise during the next year were unsuccessful, and it was only after the baby was eighteen months old and progressing strongly that finally the mother was able to diet and to regain her confidence.

The usual weight gain in pregnancy is from twenty-four to thirty pounds, and most of this is usually lost within the first two weeks after the birth. Whatever the weight gain in a pregnancy, it is unwise to diet at this time, and is not recommended.

The Conventional Approach to Obesity Following Childbirth

Conventional treatments usually include a diet programme of between 1,000 and 1,500 calories, diuretics, and appetite inhibitors. In a modern unit psychological counselling is available for the problem, although for the majority of women this is still rarely available. Careful dieting does not usually affect quantity or quality of lactation.

Recommended Remedies for Obesity Following Childbirth

1) Calc. carb.

This is a generally useful remedy for a chilly and weak person with tendencies to obesity. Everything is an effort, and pallor with sweating is frequent.

2) Phytolacca Berry
In order to curb the appetite I recommend the mother tincture, 5 drops daily.

For Obesity Associated with Water Retention

Natrum mur.
This is definitely the most efficient remedy where water retention is a problem.

For Obesity Associated with a Sluggish Metabolism

Thyroideum
This is a remedy which stimulates metabolism and elimination generally.

For Obesity Associated with Constipation

1) Bryonia
Where there is no wish to open the bowels, and the stools are small, round and hard like stones.

2) Nux vom.
Where desire to defecate is present, but ineffective. Irritability is marked.

3) Sepia
Where there is a combination of exhaustion, dragging pains, occasional severe irritability, and general indifference. Often one of the best remedies at this time.

Where the Appetite is Insatiable

1) Sulphur
When associated with excess body heat and diarrhoea.

2) Sepia
Where there is a combination of chilliness and obstinate constipation.

For Obesity Associated with Food Cravings
In all cases a strict diet low in starch and fats is necessary, together with regular exercise.

1) Natrum mur.
Craving for crisps, nuts and anything salty.

2) Lycopodium
Craving for chocolate, honey and any very sweet foods.

3) Pulsatilla
Craving for rich, creamy cakes and pastries.

Loss of Libido During the Puerperal Period

Fluctuations of libidinal level are perfectly normal throughout life for both men and women. Female libido is linked to the menstrual cycle and underlying hormonal levels, and this is part of a healthy and balanced female physiology.

Some loss of interest or diminished pleasure in sex after the birth is common to the extent of being normal. There is frequently a temporary diminished sexual desire during the post-delivery period for reasons which are not always clear or associated with any particular problems of depression. At this time the woman is focused on her own body, the recovery of her previous shape, and the health of the baby, especially if it is a first child. Anaemia, lack of sleep and new patterns of breast-feeding all make this a delicate time. What the woman needs is reassuring, non-demanding caring, and closeness and support are paramount.

Once the psychological needs of the puerperal period have been met and physical changes established, then libido is usually not a problem, and usually re-emerges quite strongly, spontaneously and naturally. Only when this lack of interest is prolonged over a period of months should it become a matter for concern and professional advice sought. In many cases the cause is unknown, but often there is a deep psychological cause relating to the actual birth, or to the quality of the woman's relationships. When the father is present at the birth, this gives support and a quality of sharing that is invaluable for the intimacy of the couple and can help to alleviate many emotional problems by fostering a depth of closeness and shared experience which may not always have been previously present.

Lack of interest in sex can of course be the result of such obvious things as the physical pain and trauma which some women experience at birth, especially when their pain threshold is at a low level. Premature or enforced sexual intercourse before the woman wants it can be both psychologically and physically painful, and healing be very prolonged. Discomfort from an episiotomy or a caesarian scar, sometimes with a stitch-abscess or a painful scar, can last for a long time, and often the least pressure causes severe pain and discomfort.

The Conventional Approach to Loss of Libido During the Puerperal Period

Tranquillizers, a variety of psychotrophic drugs, counselling and supportive therapy are all prescribed for this condition, depending upon the referring physician. Rest and avoidance of sexual activity in any forced way is usually recommended. However, many cases do not come for treatment, and the young mother too often either accepts the change in her as inevitable, or fails to believe that it is a condition that can be helped.

Recommended Remedies for Loss of Libido During the Puerperal Period

1) Arnica
Very useful when taken in the sixth potency, especially when the mother lacks energy and feels dull, and has not felt herself since the baby was born.

2) China
This is helpful where the fatigue is much more marked, to the point of almost total exhaustion. The mother needs to stay in bed and rest and has no energy or interest.

3) Pulsatilla
One of the best remedies for weak libidinal drive, changeable and mixed feelings, lack of confidence and disinterest. Heat in any form cannot be tolerated.

4) Sepia
Probably the best remedy for the problem, but to be fully effective there must usually be a combination of constipation, chill and exhaustion, irritability and feelings of indifference and disinterest.

Failure to Re-establish a Normal Cycle after the Birth
Usually the first period after the birth occurs when the baby is six to eight weeks old. If the periods fail to re-appear, the commonest cause is lactation, and it is not uncommon for the periods to be absent for several months during

breast-feeding, although ovulation and fertility are usually normal. If the periods have not returned by the twelfth week and you are not breast-feeding, then gynaecological advice should be sought. A common cause for the failure to menstruate is a subsequent pregnancy.

The Conventional Approach to the Failure to Re-establish a Normal Cycle after the Birth

After a full examination, a D&C is often recommended in an attempt to stimulate the cycle to begin again. Clomid, an ovarian stimulant, is an alternative remedy.

Recommended Remedies for the Failure to Re-establish a Normal Cycle after the Birth

1) Pulsatilla
This is usually the best remedy. It is most effective, however, when there is a combination of chilliness with intolerance of heat, absence of thirst, and a changeable weepy disposition.

2) Sepia
After Pulsatilla, Sepia is the most important remedy, with typical marked constipation, hunger and an irritable exhaustion.

3) Sulphur
Often helpful when neither Pulsatilla or Sepia seem indicated. Diarrhoea is frequent.

Ambivalent Feelings towards the Partner or Baby in the Puerperal Period

It is important to realize that ambivalence is part of life and all relationships to some degree. Everyone experiences daily fluctuations of feelings, differing only in degree and subtlety. All of us have feelings of love and hate, a need for closeness and nearness, and a need to be apart or alone. These needs for space and time apart are perfectly natural and present in everyone. The new mother needs to be accepted as she is, especially at this particular time. She needs to have her more irritable and intolerant aspects accepted and loved just as much as her more outgoing positive side. She wants her feelings to be listened to at this time, and to be treated with a degree of understanding and warmth.

There is often misunderstanding within a couple's relationship after the baby is born, and irritability because of the difficulties of communicating and sharing the ever-changing and sometimes ambivalent feelings. The new mother will almost certainly have many doubts and fears, simply because of the pressures and uncertainties of modern living. In addition to these uncertainties, a new baby can be very tiring and demanding, and an intrusion into both partners' lives because of its enormous demands and dependency. Loss of sleep, fatigue, a noisy hungry baby, can at times make the most saintly patient of mothers feel that she has had enough. Nearly all young babies make their hunger loudly known in the middle of the night as well as in the day, and this can be very exhausting on top of the fatigue of a recent pregnancy.

When ambivalent feelings arise towards the baby, a discussion of the problem with a change of routine and more help can make a lot of difference. Support and understanding from the partner is vital, as there is often a degree of unrecognized depression as a root cause. Other children can also add to the weight upon a young mother, and they must be encouraged to feel equally but differently loved and valued, and allowed to play some sort of real helping role with the new arrival. This can go a long way to reducing demands for reassurance and attention.

Sometimes a husband or partner also needs this same reassurance if he feels at all threatened. Understanding and listening are great healers, and an easy open attitude, together with as much rest and sleep as possible, can lessen a lot of ambivalence. It is essential for both partners in the relationship to feel accepted as individuals, cared for and valued enough to share intimacies which include many mixed doubts and feelings as well as straight-forward needs and positive emotions.

Another situation where ambivalence is marked is where the relationship is fundamentally a facade, held together temporarily as a matter of convenience until the baby is older or an alternative partner is free. The usually marked ambivalance is often reflected in the underlying hostility — often quite apparent unless there is a sufficiently strong bond of love and good will to work at mutual problems. The relationship has to matter enough to want to repair and mend it, otherwise separation is infinitely preferable to long drawn-out hostilities.

Childbirth is probably the major psychological event in a woman's life. Not only is she prepared for it physically and psychologically, she has also been socially and culturally groomed for if over many years. From her earliest childhood games she is exposed to the concept of babies and pregnancy, although paradoxically is usually told very little about conception or the actual birth process. Much of this important information is left either to a child's imagination, or to playground and peer-group gossip. Eventually, maybe, the real facts are clumsily and often haltingly exposed with barely hidden embarrassment by teachers or parents. This double standard only does harm and gives little reassurance to what is essentially a natural process.

Contact with other pregnant women before a woman becomes a mother herself can do a lot to foster a healthy psychological attitude. The attitude of doctors and advisors during a pregnancy is also important. At all stages, reassurance and information are needed to understand the internal structural changes and processes that occur as the foetus develops. Once the stages of the pregnancy are understood, the progress of labour, after-birth and breast-feeding should be openly discussed so that the mother, especially if she is a first-time mother, can feel less anxious and more confident in herself. It is usually the first baby and delivery that causes most psychological problems. Subsequent pregnancies usually involve far less pressure and are taken in the mother's stride, because it is not such an unknown experience and the mother has more confidence in herself.

A great fear of every mother is that there is something wrong with her baby. Usually this is unfounded, but sometimes problems can and do arise with newborn babies. I have already mentioned such a problem and the effect on the mother in the section when dealing with puerperal problems of obesity. Where there is a problem, information and knowledge is essential from the experienced child specialist or paediatrician. It is unfortunate that in many of our busy modern clinics and hospitals the doctor is all too often over-stretched and pressurized to give other than the briefest and most sketchy information. Sometimes the young mother is treated as stupid or hysterical when she is worried and demanding in any way, and information is often wrongly kept to a minimum.

When it seems that there is a problem with the health of either mother or baby, then always insist on specific information about the condition, causes and the diagnosis. Ask also about the drugs being used in the treatment and of any possible risks and side-effects. Always try to see the consultant-in-charge of the case, to clarify any problem in detail and to your satisfaction.

Every new baby makes round-the-clock demands of its mother, and because of the physical demands being made on you as a mother it is vitally important to take regular rest, together with ensuring adequate nutrition in your diet and no skimping of your own meals. Exercise and fresh air for both mother and baby are important. Partner back-up and support is the other essential ingredient. However tired he is and whatever his business and travelling commitments, his time and support are essential to the mother.

In general, the pain and exhaustion of pregnancy and delivery quickly fades into history for most mothers. The 'never again' feeling is on the whole short-lasting. For many women, pregnancy, breast-feeding and relating to the new baby all help to create a time when they are physically and psychologically at their peak. It is not uncommon for a woman to consider another child simply becuase she misses the experience of relating to a new, dependent baby as the previous baby turns into a child.

There are as many ways of responding to motherhood as there are mothers. Some women sail through every pregnancy and are always in their prime, while others are racked by nausea, insomnia and discomfort. Such variations need to be acknowledged and accepted by the woman, her partner, and the family as a whole, because they are part of life's normal variations. The conventionally 'negative' aspects of these variations are not illness or sickness — quite simply they are part of growth, development and fulfilment and maturation.

7.

INFECTIONS

Vaginitis

Vaginitis in the Pre-pubertal Girl
Vulvovaginitis is not uncommon in the young girl, and is usually due to faecal contamination. The girl must be trained to wipe herself away from the vaginal and urethral regions. Other causes are the introduction of a foreign body or the fingers into the vagina, usually an expression of the child's natural curiosity and developing sexual awareness, both of which may also cause infection. Other less common causes are thrush, bacterial infection, wearing non-cotton pants, and allergy to bubble-baths, detergents and perfumed soaps. Causes such as gonorrhoea are rare, and only occur as a result of sexual interference or assault. The other common local infections which occur are cystitis or urethritis. These are both painful and irritating, the usual cause again being faecal contamination.

Vaginitis in the Post-pubertal Girl
Vaginitis is not common as long as the hymen remains intact, the hymen acting as a barrier to ascending infection. Vaginal tampons are not infrequently the cause of infection in this age-group, and any abrasion or sore area caused by an applicator or an over-absorbent tampon can set up infection and vaginitis.

Vaginitis in the Sexually Mature Woman
The commonest infections of this age group are the sexually-transmitted vaginitis problems which only occur due to sexual intercourse. As long as

neither partner has had any contact with an infected third person, then disease of this type cannot exist, and both should remain healthy and well. If an outside contact takes place then either or both partners may be at risk even if the other person is symptom-free, since they may be a carrier without symptoms, and unaware of transmitting any type of infection.

Recommended Remedies for Vaginitis
See page 92.

Cystitis and Pyelonephritis

Bacterial infection of the bladder is one of the commonest female problems. It is particularly frequent in late pregnancy when the naturally short female urethra becomes stretched and distended by the foetus. Cystitis often occurs from bacteria originating in the anal-perineal regions, gaining access by means of a pad or a tampon string. Other causes are irritation from tight non-cotton or nylon underware and tight jeans. Bubble-baths and detergents break down the surface tension of the water, and also facilitate infection.

The usual organism responsible for cystitis is the E. Coli bacterium, which is a normal inhabitant of the large bowel. Once access has been gained via the urethra to the bladder, they can multiply rapidly. Normally there is an efficient valve mechanism at their entrance which protects reflux of urine back into the ureters from the bladder, but if this protective mechanism is in any way damaged, weak or absent, then infected urine may flow back along the ureters each time the bladder is emptied, creating a potential source of dangerous infection to the kidneys.

If the funnel-shaped urine-collecting areas of the kidney become infected, a painful condition called pyelitis — more correctly pyelonephritis — can become established. This condition is particularly common in pregnancy, and is often recurrent. There is a high temperature of 101-103°F/ 38.3-39.4°C, headache, and exhausting severe pain in the kidney area just below the last two ribs along the spinal region. Shivering rigors are common as toxin-release forces the temperature to a higher level, increasing exhaustion. The infection weakens and distorts the urine-collecting areas, which may become greatly dilated. The ureteric pathways to the bladder may become distended and tortuous.

There are other causes of bacterial bladder infection, but by far the commonest is irritation of the urethra by unaccustomed or over-enthusiastic, rough or traumatic intercourse. This is a well-known problem, commonly called 'honeymoon cystitis'. A vaginal discharge may sometimes be present near the urethral entrance and cause an ascending infection into the bladder. Other frequent causes are allergic reactions to certain soaps or a perfumed douche, a reaction to an ill-fitting contraceptive cap or diaphragm, or the excessive intake of coffee or tea.

The usual symptoms of bladder infection are of urinary frequency with the passing of urine which is felt as hot and burning. When pain is at the end of the flow, so that often only a few drops are passed from spasm, it is called strangury, and this is one of the most disagreable of all the symptoms of cystitis. Urgency is frequent with a general lack of bladder security. There is a fear of being 'caught short' as the woman often can not control an urgent desire to pass urine.

It is important for both doctor and patient to differentiate the scalding-hot pain of cystitis from the sharp soreness of urine flowing over a sensitive or cracked vulval area.

Formerly cystoscopy or visual examination of the bladder interior and intravenous X-ray pyelograms were carried out routinely and repeatedly, until the potential dangers of X-ray irradiation were recognized. Modern thinking is now quite different and much more cautious and careful. Catheterization of the female bladder is now considered potentially dangerous, because of the considerable risk of introducing infection, subsequently very difficult to control. When there is a definite problem of recurrent cystitis or pyelonephritis, then an intravenous pyelogram is probably indicated on at least one occasion to exclude the possibility of congenital malformation of the renal pelvis, which is a common factor.

The Conventional Approach to Cystitis and Pyelonephritis

Usually the woman is encouraged to take plenty of fluids. An antibiotic such as Septrin, Ampicillin and Uroleucosil or a sulphonamide is often prescribed. Often Mixt. Pot. Cit. (a mixture of Potassium citrate in solution) is prescribed to change the pH of the urine and discourage bacterial growth in the bladder. The laboratory will advise on the best antibiotic based on culture tests.

Recommended Remedies for Cystitis and Pyelonephritis

a) Cystitis

1) Aconitum
Recommended for early recent infections, often as a result of exposure to cold. Use in the first forty-eight hours when associated with a high

temperature, restlessness, and anxiety or fear.

2) Apis
For mainly urethral irritation with strangury or spasm without marked frequency. Usually very little urine is passed, and then only drop by drop. Burning and scalding pains are not a particular feature where Apis is indicated.

3) Arsenicum Alb.
Another acute remedy where there is a marked burning frequency which can be relieved by heat and warmth.

4) Cantharis
Usually the best remedy for the majority of cases where there are violent spasms of searing, lancing pain on passing water. Urgency, frequency, strangury and a constant urge to urinate.

5) Belladonna
An often used remedy where there is bladder irritation with great urgency because of burning urethral spasm, irritation and strangury. The diagnostic indicator is aggravation by the least pressure, touch or movement.

6) Pulsatilla
Recommended more for the more chronic forms with a recurrent mild and variable irritation. There is an absence of thirst and an intolerance of all heat.

7) Staphisagria
Where the cystitis is basically an irritation of the urethra from either trauma or over-enthusiastic intercourse. The pains are typically very sharp and cutting. Abstinence for a few days usually clears the problem completely, but if this is not effective, then follow with Arnica.

8) Sulphur
I use this remedy for those chronic problems that fail to respond effectively to other remedies which seem indicated.

b) Pyelonephritis (Pyelitis)

1) Aconitum
Use only in the early stages where there is renal discomfort, a high

temperature and rigors. The temperature is typically higher at night. There is usually little urine passed. The attack may follow exposure to cold, damp or trauma.

2) Berberis
One of the major kidney remedies and therefore important to consider. Weight-like kidney pains are common, tending to radiate to the back, pelvis and along the ureters. The pain feels pulling and heavy, and the sides are stiff and swollen, with a peculiar 'bubbling' quality which is specific to the remedy.

3) Causticum
Often useful in both acute and chronic pyelitis. There is a dull ache in the renal angle, typically associated with weakness and rawness along the whole renal tract.

4) Chelidonium
Although usually considered a gall-bladder remedy, this is a useful remedy with which to follow Causticum. The pain is usually right-sided, with urinary frequency and a marked yellowish-brown urine. The condition is usually improved by local heat, and pressure or movement aggravates it.

5) Dulcamara
Use for much milder cases of urinary frequency and renal discomfort, often after there has been an exposure to damp.

6) Terebintha
Use only for severe cases with the most violent spasms of burning irritation, a sense of pressure, and weight in the renal angle, with just small amounts of often blood-stained urine. The urinary frequency is typically worse at night.

Trichomonas Vaginitis
Trichomonas is a sexually-transmitted disease, involving infection by the highly mobile trichomonas organism which was first discovered in the 1940s. Trichomonas is clearly seen by a simple microscopic examination of the vaginal discharge.

Before trichomonas was discovered, all persistent vaginal discharges were often wrongly suspected of being gonorrhoeal in origin.

The major symptoms are a frothy yellow-green discharge with marked pruritus, burning discomfort or itching, usually worse before a period. The discharge has an unpleasant odour. There may be no external signs of the infection on the vulval or vaginal regions, though sometimes the area is red from the associated irritation of the labial area. Often, however, there is nothing external to see, but frequency of burning urination from the associated cystitis is very common.

The Conventional Approach to Trichomonas Vaginitis

Following microscopy of a specimen of the discharge by vaginal swab, a specific remedy is usually given. The commonest remedy used is Flagyl, which is taken orally. To be really effective, and to prevent immediate re-infection, it is essential that the remedy be taken by both partners. Side-effects are not uncommon, particularly either total intolerance or gastric upsets. The alternative which is sometimes prescribed is Pinafucin (Natomycin) in pessary form.

Recommended Remedies for Trichomonas Vaginitis

See page 92 for remedies for vaginitis, including trichomonas vaginitis.

Thrush

This is the common fungal yeast infection of the vaginal tract caused by the Candida albicans organism. Under the microscope, the fungus looks like a glistening white necklace chain — hence the medical terminology Monilia (Latin for necklace) and Albicans (Latin for white or dazzling).

Causes of Thrush

Although thrush may be transmitted by a man, it can often also be transmitted by airborne spores, so that it is not strictly a sexually transmitted disease. It is most common in mature, adult, menstruating women, especially where a course of steroids or antibiotics have recently been given. The latter have usually killed off all the normal and healthy vaginal flora and sterilized the whole tract. The normal bacterial flora of the vagina has an important role to play in keeping fungal organisms in check, and it may take several weeks before they re-form themselves again. Thrush is more common where there is diabetes present, since high urine sugar levels create an ideal environment for them to flourish and grow. It is also common in the second high-glycogen phase of the menstrual cycle under the dominance of progesterone. Thus women who are taking a high-progesterone contraceptive pill are more vulnerable to thrush infection.

Symptoms of Thrush

There is usually a rather thick, curdy, cheesy fluid discharge with marked vaginal and vulval itching and signs of external inflammation around the vulva and anal region.

The Conventional Approach to Thrush

Usually an anti-fungus treatment is prescribed such as Nystatin (Nystan) is pessary form. Another common alternative is Ketoconazole (Nizoral), which is an antibiotic. Some gynaecologists paint the uterine cervix with an anti-fungal antiseptic paint in obstinate cases.

Recommended Remedies for Thrush

See page 92 for remedies for vaginitis, including thrush.

Non-specific Vaginitis

This is an increasingly common form of vaginitis, and is nearly always sexually transmitted. The commonest organism responsible is bacterial, most frequently Corynebacterium Vaginalis.

Causes of Non-specific Vaginitis

In most cases the infection is carried and transmitted by the male sexual partner, who is usually completely symptom-free.

Symptoms of Non-specific Vaginitis

There is a thin, watery, unpleasant and greyish-green discharge with an offensive odour. In contrast to thrush, which has an increased frequency in the second (progesterone) part of the menstrual cycle, non-specific vaginitis is aggravated by high oestrogen levels, so it is commonest during the first (oestrogen) half of the cycle. It is also common during pregnancy, or when a woman is taking a high oestrogen contraceptive pill.

The Conventional Approach to Non-specific Vaginitis

Usually a course of antibiotics such as Penicillin or Tetracycline is recommended to treat the infection depending on results of laboratory tests.

Recommended Remedies for Vaginitis

Note that in the homoeopathic approach the individual causative agents are far less important than the overall symptoms of the individual. Thus the different forms of vaginitis are grouped together here by their symptoms rather than by their causes.

1) Alumina
One of the most reliable remedies for chronic problems. There is a thick and either clear or sometimes white discharge with itchy burning symptoms, always worse in the second (progesterone) half of the cycle. Vulval soreness is marked, together with often obstinate constipation.

2) Borax
Indicated where the loss is thick and gelatinous in consistency like clear egg-white.

3) Graphites
A useful and often successful remedy where the discharge is more thin and watery with a burning sensation to it.

4) Kreosotum
There is a yellowish loss, smelling characteristically of rye grain, with a burning irritation and overall weakness.

5) Merc. sol.
This is a remedy to be considered when there is an acute bacterial vaginitis with an offensive greenish-yellow thick loss, often accompanied by chilly sweating and sometimes a recurrent fever.

6) Nitric acid
The discharge is thick and cloudy, burning and excoriating. Fissuring and burning of the surrounding skin is a common symptom.

7) Pulsatilla
One of the best remedies where well-indicated. It is especially helpful in the early cycle discharges with a watery but variable yellow-green discharge, which at other times can be clear and white.

8) Sepia
This is also very helpful where the loss is offensive and yellowish, together with dragging lower abdominal and uterine discomfort. Constipation, exhaustion and irritability are marked.

9) Sulphur
Recommended especially for more chronic problems, with an offensive

discharge. There is often an associated diarrhoea, local skin eczema is common, and all symptoms tend to be worse in the mornings.

Gonorrhoea

Gonorrhoea, commonly known as clap, is a sexually transmitted disease of almost epidemic proportions, causing localized pathological changes of a strictly limited nature.

Causes of Gonorrhoea

The cause of gonorrhoea is infection by the paired bacterium Neisseria Gonorrhoea during sexual intercourse.

Symptoms of Gonorrhoea

Many women, perhaps the majority, have no symptoms at all. A slight urethritis may occur with a pus discharge from the urethra and from the surrounding infected skin rash. There may more rarely be infection of the Bartholin's gland causing Bartholinitis. The major danger to the woman is an ascending infection involving the fallopian tubes, setting up salpingitis and subsequent sterility by a process of fibrosis, blockage and contraction of the tubes. This can be a very rapid process, occurring within a few weeks of infection. Gonorrhoea can also cause blindness in the newborn baby when the mother has the disease. This is why newly born infants are often and prophylactically treated with either silver nitrate of penicillin eye-drops.

The Conventional Treatment of Gonorrhoea

Conventional treatment is effective and recommended. Either penicillin is given in one massive dose, or Tetracycline when the woman is allergic to penicillin.

Recommended Remedies for Gonorrhoea

Because of the rapidity of spread, the early and localized dangers, the virulence of the Neisseria organism once it has gained access, and the effectiveness of the conventional treatment, I do not recommend the homoeopathic approach for gonorrhoea in anything other than a secondary role. The major back-up remedies to antibiotic treatment are Medorrhinum or Merc. sol.

Syphilis

Syphilis is a notorious disease, sexually transmitted but blood disseminated. It has become increasingly common again in recent years, especially in the younger age groups, and is a far more serious illness than gonorrhoea.

Causes of Syphilis

Syphilis is due to infection by the spirochaete Treponema Pallidum. This is a long, thin, spiral-shaped, highly motile and penetrative organism, which can divide and proliferate extremely rapidly once in its ideal environment inside the cellular system of the body. The usual sites of entry are the genitalia, mouth or nipple, with a chancre or firm hard sore occurring at the point of entry, often with ulceration soon developing. When the site of entry is the cervix, the woman may be completely symptom-free and unaware of the primary infection, so that for many months she is infectious but totally unaware of it. Once the chancre develops and ulceration occurs it is literally overflowing with the Treponema organisms, and penetration soon occurs into the body. The great danger of syphilis is its high degree of virulence and activity. Within a period of ten to ninety days after infection, the spirochaetes may enter into the blood stream and thereby infect every organ of the body, including the brain. A pregnant woman may lose the foetus because of a syphilitic infection, or it may cause possible death *in utero*, abortion, or foetal damage at a key period of development, leading to congenital defects which are not discovered until the birth.

The Conventional Treatment of Syphilis

The disease can be detected and confirmed by the specific Wasserman Test on a blood sample three to four weeks after infection, and sooner by microscopic examination of the scrapings of the primary chancre. Usually a course of penicillin in high dosage is given, or when there is intolerance or sensitivity to penicillin, Tetracycline is prescribed. The whole treatment needs expert handling because of the risks involved, and should be treated by a specialized physician or clinic.

Recommended Remedies for Syphilis

There is none as effective as penicillin. As in gonorrhoea, homoeopathic remedies can only play a back-up role, and the major remedies for this purpose are Merc. sol. or Syphilinum.

Other Vaginal Infections

These include infection by Chlamydia or Mycoplasma, which are minute organisms, midway in size between a virus and a bacterium. Bacterial infection with the pus-forming organism Staphylococcus Aureus may occur as an extension of a local infection, boil or sore. Other causative organisms are still being discovered with new miroscopic diagnostic techniques.

Recommended Remedies for Other Vaginal Infections

Follow the same guidelines as in the general section for the treatment of vaginitis, page 92.

Genital Herpes

Herpes is an increasingly common sexually transmitted disease. The incidence of this condition is high and by all amounts it is on the increase globally. The origin is viral, via the common Herpes Simplex virus. There are two known types of infection. Type I (labialis) affects the mouth and lips, and is recognized by the common cold sore. Type II (genitalis) causes herpes only of the vagina, cervix and vulva. Both are highly infectious, and the oral type I can also give rise to genital infection.

Symptoms of Genital Herpes

Herpes gives rise to a variety of symptoms. Usually a cluster of small red blisters occurs in the thigh, buttock or genital areas and all or some of the blisters may form ulcerating areas which are itchy and painful. Herpes tends to be recurrent; every four to eight weeks is its usual cycle of external appearance. The first attack may be severe, and provoke a rise in temperature and tender lymph glands in the area drained from the infection. The condition is often long-lasting, and may last for months or years, the viral eruption occurring with painful regularity. Depression is common at the time of the eruption.

The Conventional Treatment of Genital Herpes

The diagnosis is made microscopically from examination of the scrapings or fluid from the blisters and ulcers. The presence of viral vesicles within the cellular tissue confirms the diagnosis.

Treatment by conventional methods is not satisfactory, and some gynaecologists would admit that there is none available. The condition has been recently given added importance because of a suggestion that there may be a causal relationship between type II genital herpes and carcinoma of the cervix. Treatment may also include the organic iodine antiseptic Betadine, or the anti-viral antibiotic Zovirax (ancylovir). Note that Herpes Zoster or shingles is quite a different and unrelated viral infection, and there is no known relationship between the two conditions.

Recommended Remedies for Genital Herpes

1) Graphites
One of the best remedies where there is a painful oozing red infected area and the fluid discharge is either clear or straw-coloured. There is itching, but little heat or burning.

2) Hepar sulph.
Oral herpes (I) is present with a typical cold sore usually in the centre of the lower lip. The upper lip is frequently swollen and tender.

3) Natrum mur.
One of our most deep-acting remedies, which has the ability to stimulate cell resistance even to viral conditions. It should be used in high potency of at least 200c. There is a very frequent cold sore eruption of the oral herpes type in the middle of either the upper or lower lips, sometimes both.

4) Nitric acid
Oral but also genital ulceration may be marked, often with cracking in the area and smarting tenderness. The ulceration especially involves the corners of the mouth and lips.

5) Psorinum
Recommended for more chronic cases, where there is weakness and chill improved by heat. Itching and infection in the surrounding area are marked.

6) Rhus tox.
There is a vesicle eruption which is itching and uncomfortable with surrounding redness. All symptoms tend to be relieved by heat and movement.

7) Sepia
Vesicles are present and feel under pressure. Redness and itching are marked,

and often ulceration of the vesicles. Irritability and constipation are frequent symptoms.

8) *Sulphur*
For chronic difficult cases where there is a burning discomfort and often a secondary infection in the area. The condition is always worse with any form of heat.

Salpingitis
Salpingitis is inflammation of the fallopian tubes or oviducts from bacterial infection.

Causes of Salpingitis
The commonest cause is an ascending inflammation from the vagina and uterine cavity into the tubes. It may occur as a complication of birth, particularly after an illegal or septic abortion where staphylococcus (bacteria organized in grape-like clusters) or streptococcus (organized in chain-like clusters) have gained entry. Inflammation as a complication of gonorrhoea is the most dangerous as well as one of the commonest causes of inflammation. The organism very quickly produces pus, distending the tubes and causing agonizing pain. It then either destroys the lining cells or blocks the tubes by fibrosis and adhesions.

Much rarer causes include complications following the specialized fallopian tube X-ray (salpingogram), or an infective complication of fitting an IUD. Tuberculosis is now a rare cause of salpingitis, at least in the West, where formerly it was one of the most frequent. Another cause is as a complication of appendicitis when abscess formation has occurred and has spread to involve the tubes. The condition needs to be differentiated clearly from acute appendicitis by the diagnosing doctor, since the latter requires immediate surgery.

Symptoms of Salpingitis
There is abdominal pain in the ovarian region which is aggravated by movement. Symptoms often include vomiting and a high temperature of 101-103°F/38.3-39.4°C. There may also be a vaginal discharge which can be purulent or haemorrhagic.

The Conventional Treatment of Salpingitis
The usual treatment is a course of an appropriate antibiotic.

Recommended Remedies for Salpingitis

1) Aconitum
Use only in the first forty-eight hours for the most acute phase, there being no specific ovarian or fallopian action of the remedy.

2) Apis
An important remedy, acting mainly on the right tube and ovary. There are severe stinging and burning lances of pain, with irritation, restlessness, absence of thirst, with little urine passed.

3) Belladonna
There is an acute infection with spasms of severe hot stitch-like pain, aggravated by the least movement or jarring. The woman is often red-faced and anxious, her temperature high.

4) Colocynth
Useful for violent and severe vice-like cramping ovarian pain, often with vomiting.

5) Lachesis
One of the most important left-side tubal and ovarian remedies, where there is an infected purulent discharge and tenderness. Tightness or pressure in any form is not tolerated.

6) Lycopodium
This remedy has an ovarian and tubal action, and is effective in predominantly mild right-sided problems.

7) Merc. sol.
Indicated where there is a high fever and a severe toxic inflammation with sweating, exhaustion and colicky pains.

8) Platina
A useful left-side ovarian and tubal remedy for the more moderate conditions. The pains are sharp and lancing, and there is often marked emotional disturbance.

9) Graphites
I use this remedy prophylactically either to prevent adhesion formation in an acute inflammatory condition, or to help reduce and break down existing adhesions when present. The remedy also has a useful left-side therapeutic effect.

Appendicitis

Appendicitis is a common acute surgical condition, especially prevalent in the younger age groups, although it can occur throughout life. There is typically pain in the lower right abdominal region, just below the umbilicus. Occasionally the pain is left-sided when the appendix is on that side and the whole of the intestinal arrangement is reversed.

Symptoms of Appendicitis

The main symptoms are a furred white-coated tongue, a moderately raised temperature, vomiting and loss of appetite. The abdomen is rigid or hard, and usually tender over the appendix area. When there is any uncertainty about the diagnosis it is often wise for a period of observation in hospital to be recommended. Doubts may occur in diagnosis when there is a possible painful salpingitis or a tubal ectopic pregnancy. A painful ovarian cystic condition of the right ovary — often a cystic and painful corpus luteum may confuse the issue and create doubt. Sometimes an exploratory operation is required when observation leaves the diagnosis still uncertain and the risks of waiting are considerable. In all cases expert care is necessary for accurate diagnosis and treatment. A serious danger to a woman in her reproductive years is of abscess formation and pus in the pelvic cavity, causing peritonitis and provoking infection and blockage of the fallopian tubes, causing sterility. This is why early and competent diagnosis and treatment are so essential.

The Conventional Treatment of Appendicitis

Surgery is necessary in all cases. Where there is an accumulation of pus, antibiotics are given to sterilize the area and prevent secondary infection.

Recommended Remedies for Appendicitis

Homoeopathy is essentially secondary to any acute surgical condition, only helping to counteract or prevent shock in the early stages and to stimulate a rapid return to normal activity after convalescence. The diagnosis and treatment of appendicitis must in no way be delayed by homoeopathic trials.

Arnica is usually the best remedy to give both before and after the operation. Post-operatively the woman may be treated homoeopathically according to any specific symptoms that require relief. For post-operative pain, Staphisagria 6 is the most effective remedy.

Rubella (German Measles)

The only real danger of rubella is to the woman in early pregnancy, because of the risks of foetal deformity, which can occur in up to 50 per cent of pregnancies where the virus has passed into the blood stream of the mother. The best treatment is prevention, either by early vaccination or by deliberate exposure of the young female child before the disease becomes a risk to her pregnancies. Vaccination after birth or in the early teens is often widely recommended.

If there has been a rubella contact in pregnancy or the mother thinks she has the infection, then antibody blood tests are recommended to identify the specific rubella antibodies present, and to measure their level of protection as well as confirming diagnosis. If the antibody test confirms that rubella is present in the first eight weeks of pregnancy, it is usually recommended to terminate the pregnancy before it develops further. Other virus agents such as varicella (chickenpox), hepatitis, influenza and smallpox may also damage the foetus in the early weeks, and when there has been a contact or an actual infection, expert advice should be sought.

Bartholinitis

The Bartholin glands are situated at the vaginal entrance, each with a duct or passage opening into the posterior wall. They function primarily as lubricating glands during sexual arousal. The Bartholin ducts are small and can be easily blocked or infected, so that abscess formation is not uncommon. The symptoms are of a very larger, painful hard and pulsating swelling at the vaginal entrance or labia. Hot baths are often recommended, or a course of antibiotics. In some cases surgical incision and drainage are required.

Recommended Remedies for Bartholinitis

1) Merc. sol.
The best treatment for acute Bartholin abscess and fever.

2) Belladonna
When the condition is hot and burning and the gland very red and tender.

3) Hepar sulph.
For milder infections and inflammatory conditions of the gland.

Bartholin Cysts

This is basically a very similar condition to the abscess, but the gland is filled with a clear cystic fluid rather than pus. Symptoms are not from infection but more from pressure, with swelling and discomfort. There is not the very severe pain, local redness or raised temperature of Bartholinitis. When the cyst is large and causes discomfort or embarrassment, it may require surgical removal.

Recommended Remedy for Bartholin Cysts

Baryta carb.
This is usually the best remedy for all but the most persistent cystic conditions.

8.

STERILITY AND FAILURE
TO CONCEIVE

Infertility may be assumed to exist if after two years of regular intercourse without contraception the woman has not conceived. Some gynaecologists put the time period as one year, but this is often too short. Many advise an opinion after one year when the woman is over thirty and after two years when in her twenties. The problem is unfortunately a common one, and as many as one in five couples now have difficulties in conceiving.

Until relatively recently it was taken for granted that the major problem was inability of the woman to conceive, and it is only recently that the clear emergence of masculine factors has changed such attitudes and made the man at least as responsible as the woman. These days both man and woman are equally involved in the investigations for infertility, and it is now realized that either male or female factors can account for 35-40 per cent of cases of infertility, the remaining 20-30 per cent being due to an incompatibility between the partners.

Female Causes of Infertility

At a Uterine Level
The lining endometrium may be damaged due to a previous infection which prevents or hinders the normal embedding process. A fibroid may distort or impinge upon the uterine cavity, and also prevent normal embedding. A uterus which is tilted or retroverted (displaced backwards) may prevent fertility; this was formerly considered to be a major factor, but is now thought to be less important. A congenital defect which is important, however, is where there is a septum or membrane across the uterus, blocking normal

development. In some cases the vaginal fluid is inadequate to transport the sperm flow or provide the fluid in which it can move to its destination.

A very important new factor is now thought to be the cervical mucous plug which normally varies with the menstrual cycle — thin, elastic and easily penetrable under oestrogen influence and at the time of ovulation, but thicker and more inelastic under corpus luteum influence and with increased progesterone secretion. When the cervical mucus is abnormally thick it may create a quite inpenetrable barrier to the sperm. Another problem in this area is that of an immune or 'hostile' reaction, with the formation of sperm antibodies which either destroy or block the passage of the sperm.

At a Fallopian Tube Level
This is one of the commonest causes of infertility, due to a blocked or scarred tube which has been damaged by infection, especially gonorrhoea, endometriosis or tuberculosis.

At an Ovarian Level
This is usually due to disease such as an ovarian cystic formation or endometriosis, which has disturbed the normal follicle and corpus luteum development. In some cases the problem is one of hormonal insufficiency, especially thought to be progesterone deficiency.

At a Central or Hypothalamic Level
Here the cause is less well understood. Often chronic ill-health, infection, shock or stress has undermined hormonal output to the ovaries, especially the output of follicle-stimulating hormone. The whole cycle of stimulation and feed-back is disturbed, and fertility suffers as a result. This is the reason why worry, tension and anxiety must be kept to a minimum during the time when the couple are trying to conceive.

Other Causes
Infertility is also related to the problem of recurrent abortion in the seventh to twelfth week. This is thought to be due to genetic or chromosomal factors, hormonal imbalance or ovarian deficiency.

Male Causes of Infertility

At a Sperm Level
The sperm is frequently abnormal in some way, usually in shape, motility

or amount. Sperm volime is reduced after infections such as adult mumps with orchitis, and can also be reduced by local heat or as a response to steroid treatments. Excess smoking and drinking is not conducive to sperm production and volume; nor is the regular smoking of marijuana. Certain environmental and occupational hazards are also sperm inhibitors, such as carbon monoxide, lead, and certain pesticides. Repeated exposure to X-ray radiation as may occur in radiology is also a sperm inhibitor. Any of the above when concentrated or continously experienced over a long period can interfere with fertility by inhibiting the level of sperm production and motility.

At a Testicular or Vas Deferens Level
This is the male equivalent to the fallopian tube level. The conducting sperm ducts or urethra may be distorted or blocked by previous or existing disease which has caused scarring. By far the commonest culprits are gonorrhoea and syphilis.

At a Psychological Level
Impotence and premature ejaculation come into this category as important and frequent causes. Stress, chronic tension and anxiety can also reduce the sperm count considerably, even when previously it has been very high.

Joint Causes of Infertility
This area of incompatibility at an ovarian-sperm level between the couple is largely unresearched and is not yet understood. The incompatibility probably exists at a chromosomal level.

Investigating Infertility

Female Investigations
These naturally vary with the individual gynaecologist or clinic concerned, and with the suspected cause of the fertility problem. A full gynaecological examination and endometrial biopsy of the glandular cells to estimate whether ovulation is occurring is usually standard procedure. It is important to estimate the thickness and elasticity of the cervical mucus, to see whether it creates a barrier or is incompatible with sperm life and motility. This is often ascertained by stretching the cervical mucus and a post-coital test, the specimen being taken within a few hours of intercourse. A specialized X-ray salpingogram of the tubes can be made, and the 'Rubin' or insufflation test can examine their function and the presence or absence of blockages.

Several direct visualization techniques of the tubes have been developed in recent years. Some gynaecologists also require direct external visualization of the ovaries and uterus by laparoscopy to estimate possible cysts or endometriosis. Temperature charts are also studied to determine the time of occurrence of ovulation, and blood assays of oestrogen/progesterone levels are usual to try to determine the regularity and occurrence of the vital ovulation. Blood prolactin levels are not infrequently requested to exclude the rare pituitary adenoma as a cause of local pressure, perhaps a skull X-ray as well to look for local displacement if suspected.

Male Investigations

These are usually less onerous than those of the woman. They include a full general and urinary check-up, and a full sperm count to estimate motility, volume and the percentage of abnormal, distorted, and otherwise non-fertile sperm. Local biopsy of testicular tissue may be required to assess the health of the testicle and its activity and sperm formation.

The Conventional Approach to Infertility

Infertility is usually classified as either primary — where no previous live pregnancy has occurred, or secondary — where there has been a previous pregnancy, although further attempts have not had the same success. In many ways conventional treatment distinguishes between primary and secondary infertility, and varies accordingly. The so called 'fertility drugs' are frequently used. Where ovulation is absent or low, the anti-oestrogen Clomid (Clomiphene) is often prescribed; it is also sometimes prescribed for the male where the sperm count is low. Pergonal or Humergon has often been used in injection form; this is a natural gonadotrophin and is used when gonadotrophin levels are reduced. Its great disadvantage is a relatively high risk of multiple pregnancy, and many gynaecologists are cautious in using it. Bromocriptine is also prescribed where prolactin production is excessively high, or Progesterone given where corpus luteum formation and functioning is inadequate or weak.

Where X-rays or direct visualization confirms a tubal blockage or scarring, or any congenital malformation of the fallopian tube or endometriosis, a D&C is often recommended, together with surgical correction whenever possible to provide a clear tube for the passage of the young ovum to the uterus without undue delay or blockage.

Before artificial insemination is considered, especially for a severe problem of premature ejaculation, some form of counselling or discussion is often recommended. Artifical insemination has wide implications, especially where the partner is not the donor, but it can often be a very successful method of pregnancy, depending on the level of blockage and malfunctioning. External test-tube fertilization with re-embedding into the maternal endometrium can also be successful, but is still at an experimental stage. The technical problems for routine laboratory fertilization and re-implantation are enormous, and for some there may be profound moral or ethical doubts about the method.

In general drugs and specialized surgical techniques are only of value where there is a very specific and accurate indication for them, otherwise they are a hit and miss method which either does not suit the constitution of the individual woman, or simply fails to work. Where there is an underlying psychological cause, the drugs often do more harm than good. Specialized counselling or psycho-therapeutic help is frequently required, either of the individual or often of the couple, particularly to avoid any suggestion that one of them is more ill or the responsible partner.

Recommended Remedies for Infertility

1) Agnus cast.
One of the best remedies where weakness, both general and of ovarian function in particular is marked. Sexual and genital development is often retarded, and sexual interest weak and slow. There is a long-standing egg-white coloured vaginal loss. Useful for impotence of the male when this is a factor in the infertility.

2) Baryta carb.
Another basic but much more general and less specific remedy for immaturity of ovarian functioning and hormonal output than Agnus cast. Useful for premature ejaculation of the male where this is a problem relevant to fertility. Weakness is generally marked.

3) Conium mac.
This remedy has a strong action on both ovarian and breast functioning. It is recommended for ovarian deficiency and is especially indicated where there is a tendency to breast tenderness and hardness. In the man, it is a valuable remedy when part of the problem is weak or partial erections and impotence.

4) *Iodium*

This remedy is usually thought of as a thyroid remedy, but it also has an important action on the ovaries, especially when the right one is tender and painful. It is a helpful back-up remedy for infertility problems in general.

5) *Lycopodium*

Useful where the right tube or ovary is affected by previous inflammation, or where the ovary is tender. Dryness is marked. This remedy is also valuable for male premature ejaculation and impotence.

6) *Nux vom.*

There is often a long history of painful irregular periods with doubtful ovarian functioning. A yellowish leucorrhoea is common, together with constipation and moods of marked irritability.

7) *Phosphoric acid*

Weakness is the main indicator of this remedy, and it is useful as a general constitutional back-up treatment or where fertility is low after a long or debilitating illness or a long convalescence. In the male both testicular output and functioning is weak, with impotence and uncertain erections.

8) *Platina*

There is sensitivity to an extreme degree of the whole sexual area, with spasm and vaginismus. The left ovary is especially tender, and overall ovarian functioning diminished. It can be a very useful remedy because of its specific genital actions. Pride is marked.

9) *Sabina*

Mainly prescribed for recurrent miscarriage of the eleventh week, but it is also recommended for infertility because of its marked uterine actions.

10) *Sepia*

Useful in the male where libido is weak and interest low. For the woman it is one of the best remedies where there are irregular periods. Yellowish leucorrhoea and painful intercourse, with dragging lower abdominal pains and general loss of sexual interest. Constipation is marked.

11) Silicea

A basic remedy, acting on the tubes and uterus, indicated especially where there is weakness or infection.

12) Tuberculinum

A good remedy where there is a history of tuberculosis of the abdominal organs, even when the original illness occurred many years previously.

9.

MENOPAUSAL PROBLEMS

The menopause marks the end of the menstrual cycle and ovulation as the reproductive period comes to an end. The age range of menopause is variable, but the span is from forty-three to fifty-five years, with an average of fifty for most women. The climateric, 'change of life' or menopause is due to hormonal changes, as was the onset of menstruation. The ovarian egg cell becomes less responsive to pituitary stimulation by the gonadotrophins, so that follicle-cell development and ovulation fail to develop. For unknown reasons many women still ovulate for about a year after the periods have stopped. Although ovum-formation and release is unpredictable and variable, it is nevertheless responsible for the unexpected pregnancies of this late time. For this reason many gynaecologists advise contraceptive caution for about a year after the last period, and a mechanical contraceptive device is recommended. The chances of conception occurring are slight — about one in 60,000 — but, they are not uncommon and care must be taken.

The ovarian production of oestrogen and progesterone reduces or stops its normal and periodic cyclical output at the menopause, but the hypothalamus often continues its production of release hormones so that gonadotrophins — follicle-stimulating (egg-ripening) and luteinising (corpus luteum forming) hormones — pour out at a high level from the pituitary. At this time the major production of oestrogen is largely taken over by the adrenal glands, and to a lesser and more variable extent by conversion from androgens within the fatty tissues of the body. Only minimal amounts are still produced by the ovaries.

The major symptoms of the menopause are hot flushes, vaginal dryness from cellular thinning, and emotional disturbances.

Hot Flushes

Hot flush is probably the most common problem, occurring usually between one and two years after the periods have stopped, although sometimes coming on before they have quite finished. It is present in 60-70 per cent of women, although only about 15-20 per cent require any treatment. There are flashes of intense heat, especially in the face and head, often spreading to involve the whole body in a sensation of overall burning heat. They last just a few seconds, coming on at any time, and are only rarely psychologically induced or triggered. The frequency varies from one or two in a day to flushing and heat every hour throughout the day and night, the woman frequently waking drenched with sweat. The face becomes red during the flush and spectacles may become steamed up from the sudden production of intense heat, which can add to the embarrassment, provoking psychologically-induced blushing and even more heat.

The cause is not really understood, although it is known to be the result of hormonal imbalance, either from low ovarian oestrogen levels or more likely from the continued and unabated pituitary output of gonadotrophins. But this does not explain the whole picture, because 20-30 per cent of menopausal women go through the entire time without experiencing any form of hot flush at all.

The Conventional Approach to Hot Flushes

This can vary considerably. Since the late 1930s when synthetic oestrogen (as Stilboestrol) was first discovered, it has been widely prescribed in an attempt to reduce the high output of pituitary gonadotrophins. In the 1960s the oral contraceptive pill was widely used and considered to be without risk. It is now prescribed far less often, and modern gynaecologists are much more concerned and cautious than their earlier colleagues because the dangers and risks are far more appreciated than in earlier days. The use of hormonal oestrogen or progesterone therapies is still largely empirical, and their effects and methods of action are not fully understood. Many gynaecologists, often at the request of their patients, no longer prescribe them.

Because many of the manifestations and symptoms of the menopause are still a matter of conjecture, and no one yet knows which symptom is caused by what area of hormonal imbalance or deficiency, prescribing is very difficult for the orthodox practitioner. An orthodox colleague, with a very balanced and overall view, recommends giving his patients Ginsing because of its known properties of naturally stimulating oestrogen production without risk, thus avoiding synthetic hormonal replacement therapy with unknown and possibly dangerous long-term consequences. Vitamin E is also often prescribed at this time, and the results are often encouraging. In general progesterone replacement therapy is felt to carry less risk than prescribing oestrogen, and it is at present the most widely prescribed hormone replacement treatment. Tranquillizers and sedatives are also widely prescribed, but they should only be used with caution as their value is limited, and their side-effects and problems are often worse than the original illness. In all cases a regular and stress-free pattern of life is advised whenever possible, with the avoidance of pressures and tension at this time.

Recommended Remedies for Hot Flushes

1) *Amyl nitrite*
Useful for sudden and unexpected flashes of heat and congestion to the head. The remedy has little depth to it, so use it for secondary or back-up purposes after the more deeper acting remedies of major importance have been prescribed.

2) *Belladonna*
One of the most important remedies for this problem, where there is restlessness, agitation, and a red, burning face, often with palpitations and great intolerance of pressure, touch or any sudden jarring or unexpected motion.

3) *Crotalus*
Only use this for the most severe cases and after Lachesis. The face is flushed almost blue with congestion, there is an associated headache, and a tendency to bleeding — either nosebleeds or a heavy uterine loss. Nearly all symptoms are worse after sleep, and the woman is restless, anxious and often weak.

4) *Kreosotum*
This is a useful intermediate remedy where there are problems of burning heat, which is always better for warmth. Unlike Pulsatilla the symptoms often spread to involve the whole body with heat and sweats.

5) *Lachesis*
For many women this is the most important remedy of all, and nearly always required at some time during the treatment. There is sweating with flushing, and often violent headaches on the top of the scalp. All symptoms are worse

in the morning, worse for sleep, and there is a typical peculiar combination of talkativeness and intolerance of any form of constricting pressure to the body, such as tight clothes around the abdomen.

6) Pulsatilla
A useful deep acting remedy for somewhat milder and very variable symptoms of flushing, always worse for heat. Apart from the face, the rest of the body may be quite chilly. Tears are almost always present.

7) Sulphur
I use this remedy in more chronic cases where there is intolerance of heat in any form, together with diarrhoea, and often infection with discharge in some part of the body.

Menopausal Dryness and Vaginal Thinning
About a third of women have this problem at the menopause. The main problem is that the vaginal surface, which throughout its menstrual life was in a constant process of change and flux under the various hormonal influences which kept it in tune, becomes less elastic and thins from its former thickness of ten to twelve cells to a thickness of only two or three cells. The original depth of cells previously supplied all the essential lubricating mucus inside the vagina during sexual intercourse, and also acted as a natural and effective protection against infection. Where thinning is severe there may be a failure to moisten at all during sexual intercourse, which due to a combination of anxiety, dryness, soreness and bleeding creates an unpleasant itching, sore condition, with burning pain and tightness. An associated vaginitis easily occurs with discharge due to infection, which is predisposed by the chaffed and easily damaged lining layer.

The Conventional Approach to Menopausal Dryness and Vaginal Thinning
In the past, oestrogen creams were always routinely prescribed and for many years considered totally safe and local in action. It is now known that this is incorrect. Like a steroid cream that is locally or topically applied, the results affect the whole body by a process of absorption and spread. Many gynaecologists no longer prescribe them, and consider them to be potentially dangerous because of a possible future cancer risk. However attractively they are packed and presented, oestrogen creams are not recommended, and if you are still using them, carefully question your doctor as to their indications

for your particular problem before continuing. The usual treatment that is now given is a simple lubricating cream or jelly such as KY, which is quite adequate for most women.

Recommended Remedies for Menopausal Dryness and Vaginal Thinning

1) Bryonia
This is the best treatment, and is usually effective. An obstinate constipation with chest weakness is a common accompaniment, often with a dry cough or sore throat.

2) Calendula
I recommend Calendula cream as the most effective local lubricating and anti-infection treatment.

3) Lycopodium
One of the major alternatives to Bryonia. The external skin is dry as opposed to the more internal or mucosal dryness of Bryonia. Flatulence, weakness and indigestion are common, the temperament being diffident, shy and nervous.

4) Natrum mur.
This is the other great remedy to consider when treating this problem. It is a very general and deep-acting treatment, and when well-indicated it is very effective. A dry cough is often present, the external skin is more waxy and greasy than dry, and it is mainly the internal mucous membranes that are affected, as with Bryonia. Emotional symptoms are always marked, with a solitary tearful depression. The local vaginal symptoms are often intensely painful.

5) Nitric acid
A far more superficially acting remedy where chaffing and rubbing has broken the nearby skin, and caused redness, cracking, splitting and sometimes infection. Pain is splinter-like and smarting.

6) Staphisagria
Another useful but more deeply acting remedy when there is painful soreness or damage to the delicate lining from sexual intercourse. Pain is considerable, and resentful feelings are common.

Flooding

For some women reaching menopause the periods become irregular, intermittent and often entirely missed for several months, only to start regularly again. Although bleeding may be almost negligible and over in one or two days, the reverse is very common, with heavy periods every two weeks or even more often. A great deal of anxiety accompanies this heavy loss, together with fatigue and frequent hot flushes. When heavy bleeding occurs at the menopause it is important to have a gynaecological checkup in every case, because it is essential to clarify the diagnosis exactly. Bleeding at this time may be due to fibroids, a uterine polyp, adenomatous hyperplasia, or excessive growth of the endometrial uterine lining. Although it is not usually the cause, cancer can never be completely excluded without a full examination.

The Conventional Approach to Flooding

Depending upon the diagnosis, a D&C is usually the treatment of choice. When the flooding is severe, hysterectomy is often recommended. Anaemia from heavy loss is corrected by oral iron replacement as indicated.

Recommended Remedies for Flooding

1) China
Often a useful remedy where fatigue and exhaustion are marked accompanying symptoms.

2) Lachesis
This wonderful and most valuable remedy is often the remedy of choice. The indications are a combination of colicy pain, usually worse at the beginning of the loss, and menstrual blood which is black, and often thick and offensive.

3) Natrum mur.
The loss is heavy and excessive, with exhaustion and tearful depression commonly present.

4) Sabina
Clots accompany the dark loss, with severe cramping pains and weakness.

5) Secale
Another valuable and deep-acting uterine remedy. There are violent cramps, the loss is dark, long lasting but with an absence of clots.

6) Sepia
One of the most useful and deep acting remedies. The periods are early and heavy, with pulling or dragging cramping pains, constipation, insatiable hunger, and often low back ache. Total loss of libido is common.

7) Sulphur
Recommended for the most chronic problems when there is an offensive loss and intolerance of heat. Sweating and an infected skin are often present, and frequently an unpleasant morning diarrhoea.

Fatigue and Tiredness
Fatigue and tiredness are common at this time, and may be due to emotional causes as much as the underlying physical reasons. The commonest physical cause is anaemia, with a jaded worn-out feeling and a general lack of interest in anything other than resting. Dizziness, pallor, palpitations and breathlessness are some of the common accompanying symptoms.

The cause of many of these disturbing symptoms may be hormonal, but because there is also a disturbed emotional state it is sometimes difficult to know what is cause and what is effect. When there is a physical problem, whether from iron deficiency or an imbalance of hormones, it must be corrected if it can be done safely and adequately. The tendency to accumulate excess body weight must also be dealt with at an early stage by dieting and exercise, before it becomes a problem.

Reassurance, understanding, explanation and a sympathetic approach from both physician and partner go a long way in helping the symptoms. Periods of rest should be encouraged at the same time as regular exercise and physical activity, so as to avoid becoming an invalid.

Emotional Problems
There is nothing intrinsically bad, weak or embarrassing about no longer having periods. It is all part of an overall pattern and should be looked upon as such. Women who have not had children, or have tried unsuccessfully for a family, are often those who feel most threatened by the end of their potentially fertile years. It is very important to stay close to your friends at this time, and women friends are particularly helpful during the

menopausal years, because they give the understanding and reassurance that can often be lacking in a marriage or partnership. Men can often be very lacking in understanding at this time, largely because of their own fears and problems, and the hormonal changes that they too must come to terms with.

Tears, depression, insomnia and anxiety are all common at the menopause, but on the whole they are short-lasting, and they do not usually constitute an illness that requires specific treatment. It is useful to be aware of the trap of over-eating to compensate for emotional needs, and it is similarly important not to indulge in excess alcohol — it too puts on weight quickly and only adds to any fatigue and sadness. Try also to avoid tranquillizers, and especially keep away from slimming pills or appetite suppressants which may lead to severe mental breakdown. I also recommend that as far as possible, and even when they are freely offered to you, you should avoid taking anti-depressants unless you are in a very severe state of depression. Like sedatives, anti-depressants are very difficult to come off when you are feeling more confident, and many provoke side-effects and dependency problems that are far worse than the original depressive symptoms.

When depression or anxiety is at all severe, or tension an unbearable problem that interferes with sleep, appetite and the enjoyment of life, then get help, but be sure that it is from either a specialist in this field or from a general physician who has sympathy and experience of emotional problems. If your depression or tension is very severe, you will need specialized psychiatric or counselling help.

Menopausal Sexuality

Unless there are severe emotional or psychological problems, there is usually little change in the pattern of a woman's sexuality at the menopause. She remains interested in sex at both a physical and an emotional level, and if there are any changes in general they are for the better, with a greater freedom of expression and enjoyment now that contraception is no longer needed. How you feel about your body relates directly to how attractive you see yourself. Negative self-imagery can undermine sexual desire far more than any hormonal changes.

Changes in oestrogen level are only relevant when there are physical problems of vaginal discomfort or dryness, or sometimes of hot flushes. The former can be very easily overcome by using a lubricant; the latter rarely interferes with sexuality. When there is a new sexual relationship at this time, perhaps after a long period without intercourse, there may be some temporary soreness or tenderness, but only if this persists should you need to seek advice. For the majority of women, sexual desire and interest does not stop at fifty, and many women feel a surge of freedom and release, so that sexual interest and satisfaction is often increased.

Obesity and ill-health are the great enemies of enjoyable sexuality. Watch your weight carefully and diet intelligently, maintaining a balanced diet which is high in fibre, minerals and natural vitamins but moderate in protein and low in starches and fats.

10.

PRURITUS VULVAE

Pruritus vulvae is the common problem of genital itching, present in every age group. Pruritus is not in itself a diagnosis of any particular gynaecological condition, but it is an important pointer in relation to other symptoms, and needs careful attention to ensure a full and proper treatment of any underlying condition.

Symptoms of Pruritus Vulvae
There is an irritation which may involve a part or the whole of the vulval area with a burning prickly type of sensation, usually intermittent and relieved temporarily by scratching. It is often aggravated by heat, and the scratching may cause bleeding or set up a local infection.

Causes of Pruritus Vulvae

Infection
The commonest cause of pruritus is either a trichomonas or monilial vaginitis infection. Women often wear very tight jeans and slacks, or underclothes made of synthetic fibre which allows no natural breathing from the skin or a passage of air to allow ventilation of sweat to be absorbed. Slight chaffing is set up, and with sweat accumulation and body heat an ideal environment is created for infection and vaginitis. Other less common causes of pruritus are genital lice or scabies, the latter less frequent than the former.

Allergy
Soaps, detergents, perfumes, deodorants, genital sprays, bubble-bath

preparations and scented or flavoured douches may all act as irritants to some women. Contraceptive or lubricant creams are common culprits, and any form of vaginal spray can set up a reaction and cause an irritation — often an allergic dermatitis with slight rash, redness and marked irritation.

Pruritus in Older Women

One of the commonest age groups to be affected by pruritus is post-menopausal women, and this is thought to be due to hormonal withdrawal, loss of body fat, and thinning of the skin in the area affected. Dryness is frequent with a burning sensation and a slight reddish rash, although the redness may be as much from rubbing as from the infection. The condition is often worse at night and may disturb sleep. Heat also tends to exaggerate the problem.

Psychological Causes

This is often an important factor, accompanying anxiety or tension, sexual fears, misunderstandings or insecurity. The psychological itching may provoke a secondary bacterial infection and complicate the condition.

Physical Irritation

Tampons or a plastic tampon inserter may set up an irritation. Perfumed tampons, although quickly discontinued, were often at fault. Any tampon that pulls or makes the skin dry may set up an irritation without the woman realizing the underlying cause, and is a danger.

Vitamin Deficiency

This is not a very common cause in Western cultures, but it is not uncommon where the diet is unbalanced or deficient. The usual factor is a lack of B group vitamins, often B_{12}.

Traumatic Causes

This includes sexual interference or rape, where there may be a combination of induced vaginitis and psychological trauma playing an important role in the pruritus.

Other Causes

In a long-standing and neglected case, cancer of the vulval skin may cause a thickening; with an itchy irritation of the vulval area. Diabetes, with a high urinary sugar content, can sometimes set up a local infection.

The Conventional Treatment of Pruritus Vulvae
Where diabetes is suspected as an underlying cause, urinary and blood samples to ascertain sugar levels are necessary. A scraping of the skin in the area is frequently taken to examine the health and depth of the cellular layers and to clarify the diagnosis, as with scabies or some of the skin diseases. Threadworm infection can be seen from a swab and the infestation treated accordingly.

In many cases hydrocortisone or steroid creams are prescribed for pruritus. Betnovate (Methasone valerate) is often given, and usually serves to keep the condition chronic and just beneath the skin, but it does not cure it. Oestrogens or progesterones have been prescribed in a variety of forms in an attempt to balance hormonal deficiencies. Antibiotics like Neomycin or antihistamines such as Synalar are often given when there is an actual or suspected infection. Where the infection is severe, some doctors recommend the local injection of 95 per cent alcohol in an attempt to numb the area and reduce the itching sensation. Tranquillizers and sedatives are also commonly used, as too are iron and vitamin pills.

Recommended Remedies for Pruritus Vulvae

1) Belladonna
I only recommend this remedy when there is very marked redness and itching heat with pronounced sensitivity to touch. Belladonna is best for recent cases.

2) Caladium
Recommended as one of the best specific remedies providing that there is not an underlying physical cause of any kind, which must always be corrected first. Caladium is extremely helpful in most cases, especially where there is a creeping sensation under the skin and severe itching, which is always worse at night and with heat. Insomnia may be a problem.

3) Calendula
I recommend Calendula cream locally as the best application to use to relieve the symptoms, but the remedy must be accompanied by oral treatment in all but the mildest cases.

4) Cantharis
I use this remedy when burning itching is the worst symptom. There is a sense of having been 'scalded', and the skin feels quite raw.

5) Psorinum
Useful for more chronic irritations, especially of the elderly, often associated with an offensive discharge and infection in the region.

6) Rhus tox.
Indicated where there is an itchy red eruption requiring constant scratching, which is usually relieved by local heat.

7) Sulphur
A major remedy for the condition with redness, itching, eruptions and infection common. The condition is nearly always aggravated by water and by heat.

8) Urtica
This remedy is useful for a stinging itching condition with local vesicle or bleb formations.

11.

PROLAPSE AND LEAKAGE

Prolapse

Prolapse is nearly always due to damage at childbirth, although in most cases the symptoms only occur many years later, notably after the menopause. Uterine prolapse is usually associated with weakness or prolapse of one of the adjoining organs.

Prolapse is when the uterus drops down from its normal position within the pelvic cavity to a lower abnormal position. For convenience it is classified into three major types or degrees of severity. First degree prolapse is when the uterus herniates into the vaginal cavity. Second degree prolapse is when the uterus drops further and appears at the vaginal orifice. Third degree prolapse is when the uterus has dropped right down and appears completely or to some extent outside the vagina (procidentia). As the uterus herniates or descends, it almost inevitably drags with it the closely associated bladder, causing urinary symptoms.

Causes of Prolapse

In most cases damage to the pelvic floor of supporting muscles and ligaments is due to a prolonged and excessively strained labour. Forceps may have added to the damage, as may a precipitate birth with a too rapid appearance of the head. Multiple pregnancies or a particularly large foetus may have been the final factor, and aging, heavy lifting and strain give rise to more pressure. After the menopause the supporting muscles, ligaments and fibrous tissues become weaker, and they lose tone and resilience, especially if they have previously been stretched, torn, damaged or weakened. The other frequent cause is obesity, with a general decline of fitness and exercise.

Chronic smoker's cough or a bronchitic condition can also severely weaken the pelvic area.

Symptoms of Prolapse

Apart from the external appearance of the dropped uterus, which is not usually an early symptom, the commonest sensation is a feeling of everything dropping down inside. There is a dragging discomfort often associated with bladder disturbances, as it too becomes involved in the displacement. Frequency of urination is common, with leakage when laughing, coughing or sneezing. Vaginal discharge may occur from infection as the normal defence mechanisms are interfered with. Fatigue and exhaustion are common, together with backache, pain from ulceration, and pain during sexual intercourse. There is usually marked relief from lying down.

The Conventional Approach to Prolapse

A ring pessary to support the pelvic floor is commonly prescribed for mild cases. For other cases surgery is usually recommended. A colporrhaphy is a surgical repair or 'darn' of the weak pelvic floor, though if this is not possible or the area too extensive, then hysterectomy is usual.

Commonly Associated Forms of Pelvic Organ Prolapse

Prolapse of the Bladder (Cystocoele)

This is generally less common than uterine prolapse. Where uterine prolapse is severe, the bladder is also dragged down, as occurs in procidentia. Part of the bladder drags or bulges into the vaginal wall, putting pressure on the area and causing discomfort with bearing-down vaginal pains, and a tendency to recurrent cystitis or urinary leakage.

Prolapse of the Urethra (Urethrocoele)

The urethra sags, or is distorted and kinked, and appears below the pubic area, losing its normal supported relationship to the bladder and vagina. Severe urethral irritation and urinary frequency are often the consequences.

Prolapse of the Bowel (Rectocoele)

Weakness in the posterior vaginal wall allows the rectum to bulge through the posterior vaginal cavity, sometimes interfering with a normal bowel action because of pain or discomfort. Unless the rectum is manually replaced through the vagina, it may be impossible to have a normal bowel movement.

Prolapse of the Vagina (Enterocoele)

In this condition the weakness does not involve the uterus or surrounding organs, and only the vaginal walls are involved with the organ doubling up into itself, creating pain and discomfort.

Prolapse of the Ovary

In this condition, not uncommon after hysterectomy, the ovary drops down into the vacant space formerly occupied by the uterus, due to lack of support by the normal ovarian ligaments which hold it in place. There is pain and discomfort, especially during sexual intercourse.

Recommended Remedies for Prolapse

1) Aletris far.
This is recommended as a specific by some practitioners. Use it after the other major deep-acting remedies rather than beforehand.

2) Belladonna
Indicated where burning heat and spasms of pain come with severe irritation and dragging discomfort. Redness and local inflammation are often marked.

3) Natrum mur.
Indicated where there is marked weakness with heavy dragging pains, and the woman has to sit down to stop the uterus from prolapsing. In general the condition is improved by local firm pressure.

4) Nux vom.
Indicated where the condition is marked by spasms of sudden pain, and discomfort and irritability are marked.

5) Pulsatilla
Useful in milder problems with typical weakness, tears and intolerance of heat.

6) Secale
Especially valuable where the bladder is also involved.

7) Sepia
Often the best and deepest acting remedy.

Leakage

Leakage, also known as stress incontinence, usually occurs in the post-menopausal woman, and is associated with prolapse in one form or another. In about 50 per cent of cases the condition is due to a simple bladder herniation or cystocoele without uterine prolapse being present. The commonest cause is strain from an ill-conducted labour or from a series of multiple births. The bladder descends into the vaginal region, with a distortion of the urethra.

In the past mothers were left in labour for far longer periods than is now usual, the only criteria for intervention was foetal rather than maternal health. Fortunately such attitudes are changing, and mothers are no longer left for long periods to strain ineffectively, causing weakness, exhaustion, and later problems of depression and fear.

Symptoms of Leakage

The major symptom is slight bladder leakage from any sudden movement, change of position, or coughing, sneezing, laughter or hiccup.

The Conventional Approach to Leakage

In general the best treatment is prevention, by avoiding unnecessary prolonged labour or forceps delivery unless it cannot be avoided. It is often better to carry out an early elective caesarian section for both the mother's and the baby's health, than to allow the mother to get into an exhausted state. Early episiotomy is also required, and more spacing out of pregnancies is recommended when couples plan a large family. Orthodox treatment of the condition is surgical, by a repair or colporrhaphy, as a ring pessary is rarely effective.

Recommended Remedies for Leakage

1) Causticum

The most important of the remedies for leakage because of its strong tonic bladder action. There is an involuntary spurt of urine when coughing or sneezing.

2) Ferrum phos.

Another valuable remedy where there is a combination of bladder irritation, urinary frequency and urgency, and loss of a few drops of urine if the woman is 'caught short'.

3) Natrum mur.
Very valuable when carefully prescribed. There is a lack of urinary confidence, often going back over many years. There may be spasm and blockage, and an inability to pass anything in the presence or closeness of others. Dryness, sadness and irritation are often also marked.

4) Pulsatilla
Use Pulsatilla where there is weakness and often a slight loss of urine when sitting or from fear or laughter. The whole area is weak and often unreliable. Heat cannot be tolerated in any form and tears are never far away.

5) Scilla
This is a more locally acting remedy to be used for back-up support to the other major remedies if they are not giving satisfactory results.

6) Sepia
Often valuable because of its action on the uterus and associated organs, and valuable for prolapse in the genital area. Constipation is marked.

7) Zincum met.
The bladder is weak, slight urinary losses are common, and fidgety restlessness is marked.

12.

GENERAL BREAST PROBLEMS

The diagnosis of a breast lump depends on many factors, and it is important whether the lump is painless or causes discomfort. The most frequent causes of a painless breast lump are adenoma, a simple cyst or cancer. A painful and tender lump may be caused by fibrocystic disease of the breast tissue, a periductal mastitis, or an infection. It is particularly important to exclude and diagnose any cancerous condition at an early state, and early diagnosis depends on regular self-examination and initiative.

Painful Breast Lumps

Fibrocystic Disease
In this condition the breast tissue is coarse or lumpy with areas of glandular enlargement. The breast is tender and feels heavy with discomfort, particularly in the outer areas — the axillary tail or armpit area of the gland is particularly painful to touch and usually worse before a period. There are two types of the condition which are well-recognized — a nodular or more diffuse form, and a cystic form with small local swellings which appear and vanish with the phases of the cycle. The condition is common, and often occurs in women in their late twenties and thirties. The cause is unknown, but it appears to be associated with hormonal imbalance, especially with high oestrogen and low progesterone levels. It is often aggravated by the oral contraceptive pill, is worse just before a period, and better during pregnancy and after the menopause.

The common treatment is to give one of the anti-prostaglandin drugs, because these are increasingly thought to play an important role in the cause of the pain. Drugs such as Naproxen or Danazol are frequently prescribed. To date there are no known risks from their use, but if you are taking them, do keep abreast of the latest information about them. Anti-prolactin drugs are also often prescribed because high prolactin levels are also thought to be a cause, and progesterone therapy is sometimes given in an attempt to replace the hormone. A multiple approach is common when the diagnosis is uncertain or unknown, and to some extent the patient is at risk from such a hit and miss approach. More conservative treatments include the reduction of tea and coffee intake because of their high xanthine content, and to give the harmless B vitamins, and diuretics to eliminate fluid retention. Tranquillizers are commonly given to relax the patient and to raise the pain threshold. A well-fitting bra goes a long way to give support and some relief from pain.

Recommended Remedies for Fibrocystic Disease

1) Belladonna
Where there is an acute and hard tender swelling of the breast with great tenderness and sensitivity to the least movement or jarring, aggravated by being caught off balance. There are spasms of tearing and darting pains in the breast. Heat is often marked with the pain.

2) Bryonia
There is less heat and acute pain, but the breast feels much more hard and heavy. The condition worsens with every period.

3) Carbo animalis
For right-sided problems where there is a hard and painful nodule with spasmodic pain. The skin over the lump has a bluish-violet discolouration.

4) Conium
One of the best remedies where tenderness is marked before the period, the area feels hard, and particularly where the right breast is involved.

5) Lapis albis
Indicated for a painful nodule which feels hard, with burning spasms of pain.

6) Plumbum
Useful where the whole breast is firm and painful with tenderness,

accompanied by very severe and obstinate constipation.

Periductal Mastitis

Periductal mastitis is the other common cause of a painful and tender breast swelling. The problem is an inflammatory swelling of an area of the milk duct, usually just under or near to the areola, which is most frequent in the inner segment or lower area of the breast. The swelling is not affected by the cycle and it is often aggravated by local pressure or cold.

Periductal mastitis needs to be differentiated carefully from another painful inflammatory condition called costochondritis which occurs in the costochondral junction of the ribs and the breastbone. This is a skeletal problem rather than a glandular one, though it creates a painful lump that seems to be in the breast. It is usually clearly diagnosed by the extreme tenderness of the joint, and it is clear that the swelling is within the joint and beneath the breast glandular tissue. The problem is also common in men, who often wrongly associate such severe local pain as being of cardiac origin.

For periductal mastitis, surgery is usually recommended. Costochondritis is treated by reassurance, analgesics or painkillers, and sometimes by the local injection of anti-inflammatory agents, often of the steroid type.

Recommended Remedies for Periductal Mastitis

1) Belladonna
Where there is heat, redness and sensitivity of the entire breast area, with marked redness of the overlying skin and sometimes bouts of high body temperature.

2) Graphites
There is hardness and obstruction of the mammary duct with inflammation and tenderness. It is one of the best remedies, especially where the woman is too heavy, chilly and usually constipated. In general the breasts are tender and hard before as well as after the periods.

3) Hepar sulph.
I recommend this remedy after Belladonna for longer and more drawn-out conditions of inflammatory blockage.

4) Merc. sol.
Only recommended where the condition is most acute, without the burning of Belladonna, but with marked sweating and often a generalized toxic reaction. Diarrhoea is common.

5) Phytolacca
Probably the best general and most important remedy to consider. The lump is painful and tender, and there is an inflammation which is always aggravated by chill, damp or disturbing emotion.

6) Sulphur
I recommend this for chronic conditions which are not responding to other seemingly well-indicated remedies.

Painless Breast Lumps

Simple Cyst
This is one of the commonest causes of the isolated breast swelling, and is found in all age groups. The cause is largely unknown, but it is not associated with fibrocystic disease or related to obvious hormonal or menopausal cycle changes. The lump is usually small, freely mobile, and is often discovered by accident at a routine check-up or by self-examination of the breast area. It has no symptoms other than its presence, gives rise to no discomfort, and it cannot be seen from the surface. It may vary in size from time to time, but not clearly with the cycle. The diagnosis is usually made by aspiration and the presence of a clear fluid. It must be clearly differentiated from cancer, and this is usually confirmed by a mammogram or specialized breast X-ray, and often by biopsy and microscopy of the cells, including any present in the clear cystic fluid.

   Accurate diagnosis of the condition is essential. It can then be aspirated from time to time, removed surgically if the woman wishes, or can just be left and observed.

Recommended Remedies for the Simple Cyst
Homoeopathic treatment is only recommended when the diagnosis has been clearly made and any cancerous condition has been thoroughly excluded.

1) Baryta carb.
Recommended as a general remedy for painless cystic breast swelling,

although Baryta does not have a specific mammary action.

2) *Calcarea*
More deeply acting than Baryta, where there is often an underlying genetic or constitutional problem. The woman is large, flabby, pale and chilly, her breasts are heavy and fatty, and she is exhausted and perspiring. The lump is a single swelling which can be in either breast and is without pain or tenderness.

3) *Conium*
This is a specific breast remedy and is strongly recommended. The single cyst is usually right-sided, hard and mobile.

4) *Phytolacca*
The other great specific breast remedy, useful for more tender but painless cystic conditions.

5) *Iodium*
Often valuable where the breasts are smaller but still flabby, without much fat or glandular tissue. There is a single simple cystic swelling, without much pain or tenderness.

6) *Silicea*
Recommended for the chronic cystic swelling where the breast is small or withered, and the lump often long-standing and of an inflammatory origin.

Breast Adenoma
This is in many ways similar to the simple cyst except that it tends to be firmer, contains no fluid, and does not vary in size. It is a small localized benign tumour called a fibroadenoma, which is a ball of fibrous and glandular tissue of unknown origin. It presents itself as a firm, round, smooth and very mobile little swelling without tenderness. The diagnosis is made by biopsy and X-ray mammogram to exclude cancer, and it can easily be removed surgically by a small local operation.

Breast Cancer
This is now a common condition, most frequent around the menopausal years, and affects up to one in fifteen women. The best treatment in every case is early diagnosis and surgery, because at present prevention is not

possible. Any painless lump must be treated with suspicion by all women, and although by far the majority of lumps prove to be benign — either a cyst or adenoma — at least 20 per cent of cases are malignant and need urgent attention. Proper diagnosis by a physician or gynaecologist with expert knowledge is vital.

Regular monthly self-examination of the breasts, feeling each quadrant, including the areola and nipple carefully, is vitally important, as is annual gynaecological screening including a pap smear test and a mammogram for all women in the reproductive age-group. If in doubt about a swelling, a tender area, or a change in the breast, get a specialized opinion. Where there is a family history of breast cancer the risks are far greater, and a woman with that background should be particularly careful about any isolated painless swellings or lumps. The cause of breast cancer is still unknown, although there are many theories. Because the causes are not understood there is unfortunately no known prevention, and early diagnosis is at present the only safe answer. Surgery — mastectomy — is the best treatment, with no other real alternatives, and the success rate is about 90 per cent. In some cases radiotherapy is required, and sometimes a course of cytotoxic drugs to follow.

Recommended Remedies for Breast Cancer
Homoeopathy is not the best treatment for cancer of the breast, although several remedies are known and sometimes recommended. In general it is a mistake to delay matters by trying homoeopathy where surgery gives such good results and where waiting can allow a far more serious condition to develop. Homoeopathy should only be used as a back-up treatment to surgery and excision of the growth. Surgical techniques and results are improving all the time in this area, and supported by homoeopathic preparations and after-care there should be an uneventful recovery.

Problems of Breast Size

The Breasts are Too Small
A great deal of insecurity often centres around the size of a woman's breasts. The belief that her breasts are the 'wrong' size can cause deep feelings of inadequacy and lack of confidence.

There is no such thing as a normal size of breast, and breasts come in many shapes and sizes. As well as this variety, a woman's breasts change constantly from pre-puberty to the menopause. Small breasts are not unattractive or asexual, and media persuasion can do a lot of harm in suggesting that there are attainable ideals of breast size and shape. I have seen women pressured and undermined by their partner to have cosmetic surgery because the man concerned needed a woman with large breasts to realize some of his own fantasies.

Most of the results I have personally seen of cosmetic breast enlargement have been unsatisfactory, and have often been a disaster. Scarring is often unsightly, and the implants have sometimes collapsed, moved, needed replacement or become infected, all of which needed further incisions and more scarring. Most of the women I have seen ended up far less confident and more depressed than before. In retrospect few of them would recommend cosmetic surgery.

Recommended Remedies for Small Breasts

1) Baryta carb.
The breast is flat from loss of glandular tissue.

2) Conium mac.
Useful where there is a degree of soreness and tenderness which accompanies the diminution in breast size.

3) Iodium
A general remedy to consider where there is loss of glandular tissue, and flattening of the breast without pain.

4) Silicea
Where the breasts are small and flat without any recent loss of tissue; they have always tended to be small, and the body is often thin or undersized.

5) Tuberculinum bov.
Useful when there is a combination of weakness, exhaustion and pallor with loss of flesh in the breast area. A dry hacking intermittent cough and general chest weakness are usually present to confirm the diagnosis.

The Breasts are Too Large
This is an equally sensitive area, where too often the woman feels vulnerable but doesn't like to bother her G.P. with the problem. In many ways it is more easily dealt with because it is usually associated with a weight problem,

a great deal can often be done by sensible, regular dieting. A strict programme of exercise is recommended, with specific exercises to firm the whole breast and pectoral area so that the underlying muscles and tissues can tone up and any retained fluid in the area be eliminated or redistributed. The whole process takes about six months, and during this time it needs the confidence of the patient to attend regularly. Excessive weight on the hips, abdomen and buttocks is associated, and only very rarely is breast development excessive whilst the rest of the body is slim. Although the conventional approach in some cases is reductive surgery, especially where the condition is localized to the mammary glandular tissue, in general it is not recommended other than for exceptional problems.

Recommended Remedies for Large Breasts

1) Calcarea
Where the breasts are enlarged and heavy, and the woman is chilly, pale and very exhausted.

2) Conium
Indicated when there is excess glandular development with pain and tenderness.

3) Natrum mur.
Recommended as a treatment where fluid retention is marked in the breasts as well as in the body generally.

4) Sulphur
Swelling, irritation and sensation of heat are common symptoms, together with sweating and discomfort in the breast area.

13.

FIBROIDS

A fibroid, or more correctly a myoma, is the commonest simple growth of the uterus occurring in the menstruating woman. The lump is not predominantly one of fibrous tissue, but is made up almost entirely of muscle cells, and is surrounded by a fibrous capsule which encloses it within the uterine wall. These growths may be single or multiple, and can vary considerably in size, from the size of a pea to the size of an orange. Less than 1 per cent of fibroid growths become cancerous and break through the surrounding capsule to infiltrate the uterus, and fortunately this is not often seen. They are very common — about one in five adult women over thirty-five have fibroids in one form or other, especially those who have not borne children.

There are four common positions for fibroids to occur: the intramural fibroid is the commonest variety, lying within the muscle wall of the uterus; the subserous fibroid lies more on the surface of the uterus; the submucous fibroid is almost within the cavity and beneath the lining endothelium; finally, cervical fibroids do occur, but are very rare.

Causes of Fibroids
The cause of fibroids is unknown, but they are believed to relate to oestrogen activity, since they tend to increase in size in women on high oestrogen contraceptives as well as during pregnancy, and usually get smaller after the menopause.

Symptoms of Fibroids
Often there are no symptoms at all, depending upon the position within

the uterus. When the fibroid is large it produces more of a sense of discomfort than a pain. The commonest symptom is usually menorrhagia or heavy periods, with flooding or clots due to irritation and engorgement of the endometrium. Sometimes there is a chronic leucorrhoeal or mucous discharge throughout the cycle. When there is heavy bleeding, it is usually worse on the second and third days. The common problem is congestion of nearby regions, so that colicky period pain or dysmenorrhoea may occur, together with frequency of urination or recurrent cystitis from bladder irritation, or delay in passing either water or faeces from pressure blockages. Recurrent miscarriage is one of the most severe and serious symptoms, and a reason for surgery. The flooding may cause such heavy losses that anaemia develops with weakness and dizziness.

The Conventional Approach to Fibroids

A D&C is usually recommended initially, together with a hysterogram or specialized X-ray outline of the uterus cavity to ascertain any displacement or distortions. In making the diagnosis the physician must very carefully exclude other similar problems, especially ovarian cyst, endometriosis, pregnancy, and cancerous growth.

There are two conventional treatments, and both are surgical. The first is local removal of the myoma or myomectomy, when the fibroid is not large or causing severe pressure symptoms. The other alternative is hysterectomy, when the whole uterus and myoma are removed together. Unless there are any very severe problems or contraindications the fibroid is best removed locally, but where a fibroid has grown rapidly in a short time, this may be an indication for a hysterectomy in view of the slight but significant risk of malignancy.

Recommended Remedies for Fibroids

1) Aurum mur.
The uterus is markedly enlarged, and the periods are heavy, often with a yellowish leucorrhoeal discharge throughout the cycle.

2) Belladonna
Useful when there is severe and heavy flooding with a bright red loss and clots, with extreme sensitivity to sudden movements or to touch.

3) Calc. iod.
One of the best local remedies which gives very good results when the fibroid is not large and not causing very heavy losses. There is a colicky dysmenorrhoea just before the period is due.

4) Fraxinus amer.
This is sometimes recommended as a specific for the condition, but I generally prefer to use Calc. iod.

5) Lachesis
This can often prove useful, especially for general problems of uterine congestion.

6) Phosphorus
This is a specific remedy where there is a heavy loss of bright red blood.

7) Sepia
I use Sepia or Lachesis, as a back-up remedy for uterine congestion.

8) Silicea
Another specific for small but recurrent fibroid problems.

9) Tarentula hisp.
Useful where there are very severe large fibroids with a lot of pain, heavy loss, and restlessness.

14.

CANCER

Although homoeopathy cannot effectively treat cancer, part of its overall approach is the discussion of areas of possible concern for every patient, to inform, to allay anxiety, and most importantly to foster early awareness, diagnosis and treatment.

Until recently the most terrifying diseases were plague, syphilis and tuberculosis; now it is cancer, followed closely by coronary thrombosis. The exact causes of cancer are still not yet known in spite of several decades of research, tests and theory. It may be that we are in fact looking at several diseases and not just one. It seems likely that the eventual cause will fall into a combination pattern of micro-infection, a transmitted element and a genetic predisposition, both treatable and preventable, but until this is clarified, the disease remains a frightening one and, just like its predecessors, shrouded in mystery and speculation.

Cancer is the end result of what in most cases is an undetectable pre-cancerous process of local irritation, often over a prolonged period. During this pre-cancerous period a group of cells change their developmental pattern and appearance to become cancerous. When this change happens, these cells start to divide abnormally, get out of control, and invade surrounding tissues rather than working in harmony with them. There is no longer a partnership or symbiosis with surrounding groups of cells, and the cancer rapidly grows to spread by every possible channel, including the blood stream and lymphatics, to infiltrate, penetrate and destroy its own cellular kind. When a growth or tumour develops but remains enveloped or encysted within a wall of fibrous tissue, causing pressure but not breaking through into the neighbouring regions, then it is called benign. When it is invasive and spreading, knowing no boundaries, then it is malignant or a cancer. One in fourteen of all women develop cancer in some form during their lifetime. The commonest cancer sites for women are the breasts (25 per cent of cases), ovaries (25 per cent), uterus (14 per cent), and cervix (2 per cent), though it can occur anywhere in the body. In general, cancer of the breasts and cervix occur in younger women who are still menstruating, and uterine cancer tends to develop in the older post-menopausal woman.

Known or Suspected Pre-cancerous Factors

Chronic Irritation
Chronic irritation or constant rubbing over a long period in certain areas of the body forms a horny fibrous layer, which if continued to be irritated may in some cases eventually turn malignant. Similarly any large ulcer or lesion may develop a malignant centre to it if it is constantly irritated over a prolonged period of time.

External Irritants
Exposure to a variety of potentially toxic chemicals, tars, tobacco, asbestos or herbicidal sprays may cause cancer from prolonged tissue irritation over a long period, and this is often only recognized in retrospect. There are also other environmental hazards and pollutants which are a matter for concern and may be carcinogenic, especially high levels of lead and carbon monoxide in our cities, and more globally the toxic radioactive cobalts and DDT, which have become distributed to every corner of our planet.

X-ray Irradiation
Frequent exposure to X-rays is a cancer risk, and any form of radiation may be dangerous, including excessive sunlight. Every television set has its risks because of the low but significant output of X-ray irradiation, and for this reason it is not recommended to view from a position too close to the screen for long periods.

An increasingly recognized factor is any exposure to highly radioactive atomic fall-out and nuclear waste, with a high incidence of leukaemia and cancer among workers in the nuclear power and weapons industries.

Hormones
The role of hormones in cancer formation is still unproven, but is suspected, especially in female cancer. Oestrogen is especially suspect in setting up

the environment for a pre-cancerous condition to develop and is best avoided over long periods whenever possible.

Trauma
Trauma has sometimes been associated with cancer formation, and a knock or blow to the breast is sometimes been thought to be a possible cause of breast cancer, creating an area of fibrosis or infection. Most authorities now consider it to be a rare cause, more feared than real, and believe that most accidents and traumas heal without latent cancerous trouble.

Blockage
Blockage or removal of natural drainage are a possible pre-cancerous risk. For reasons which are not yet understood, a cancer may sometimes develop many months later, seemingly when toxic reabsorption sets up an irritating focal point elsewhere in the body.

Genetic Factors
Cancer is not inherited in any direct way, but there may be an increased genetic predisposition where cancer has occurred in a family, and this is especially true of breast cancer. Where there is a history of this disease in the family you should be especially careful, and make regular monthly self-examinations of the breasts. Have an early second opinion if in any doubt about a possible lump or swelling.

Diet
There is little direct evidence of dietic involvement, although high coffee intake is reported in the United States as being statistically linked with cancer, especially with carcinoma of the head of the pancreas, which twenty years ago was one of the rarest of all tumours and is now one of the most common. A diet low in essential proteins, vitamins and minerals may also pave the way for malignant formation.

Psychological Factors
Last but by no means least, it is likely that an unhealthy psychological attitude may be an important factor in providing the state of mind for cancer development.

Genes
Recent research studies on oncogenes and viral links look likely to offer

promising treatment developments over the next few years.

Symptoms of Cancer

There is usually a lump or swelling which is often quite painless. There may sometimes be an unusual or inexplicable discharge or bleeding. Other possible symptoms include a change in size of an area of the body, or a difference in normal functioning and rhythm, especially of the bowel, digestion and appetite, or urinary patterns. There may also be an inexplicable loss of weight.

The Conventional Approach to Cancer

As prevention at the time of writing is impossible we have to rely on early diagnosis and surgery as the best methods of cure, with homoeopathy playing a very secondary background role in most cases. Increased sophistication in cellular microscopy has allowed doctors to recognize the condition in its earliest pre-cancerous phases, before there is active infiltration and growth into nearby tissues. Treatment can therefore be initiated very early, and well before there are any symptoms. This is especially available for cervical cancer by means of the pap smear test which should be a regular annual measure for all adult women. It is likely that such early diagnosis will soon be available for other areas of the body. Regular self-examination with annual checkups by a specialist gynaecologist or in a 'well-woman' centre are recommended. For surgical treatment to be successful, it is essential that the cancer be detected before it has 'seeded' or generalized. With early diagnosis there is an 80 per cent recovery rate from breast cancer. Radiation of the area or chemotherapy with cellular toxic drugs may also be required if the growth has spread more widely.

Where cancer of the uterus is suspected, a D&C is often required as a first investigation, with microscopy of the cells and usually a biopsy of the affected area. Where a breast is the site of the suspected cancer, the usual treatment is aspiration of any fluid, microscopy, and a biopsy of any lump which is suspicious. Where the cervix is involved, investigations include a pap smear test for microscopy, and direct visual examination of the area which may be affected. Where cancer of an ovary is suspected, the investigations are somewhat different. An exploratory operation is often required, with a visual examination or laparoscopy of the ovarian area and surrounding abdominal cavity. Pelvic ultrasound examination can now give valuable information about ovarian health.

The Psychology of Cancer

The thought of mutilation by operation, and especially the loss of a breast, is very worrying for most women, as associated with irreversible damage to her self-image and her sexuality. Cancer conjures up images of depression and despair, prolonged illness, pain, incapacity and dependence. Such feelings are often at their height when the disease is first suspected or diagnosed, and the reality of the situation has not yet displaced long-feared fantasies. Once treatment has been initiated and a full and proper diagnosis made, the woman can often begin to relax a little and let the experts take over the job. Once a therapeutic team has been formed and the woman feels part of it, able to ask questions and be more of an observer, she immediately feels better and more hopeful.

At present there is no known way of preventing cancer other than avoidance of exposure to known or suspected cancer irritants. Keeping health and fitness to a high level with regular exercise and avoiding excess strain and fatigue whenever possible are very important. The best psychological attitude is one of not bottling things up, not being excessively ambitious, and enjoying relaxation and pleasure to the full. Whenever possible, stress should be kept to a minimum, although a certain degree is naturally unavoidable in our society. The avoidance of excesses includes not taking in too much alcohol or tobacco. Cigarette smoking over a long period is a proven cause of cancer, and when combined with the high-oestrogen pill in young women can be very risky. The combination of cigarette smoking and the oral contraceptive pill over the age of thirty is especially dangerous and should be avoided without prolonged delay.

Cancer is curable, and this has been proved innumerable times, but as with any illness the curing of cancer depends upon early diagnosis. If you are in any doubt whatsoever, get an opinion, and if still in doubt get others until your mind is at rest.

Finally, however homoeopathically orientated you are and whatever remedies you are using or being prescribed for the condition, they must not hold up or interfere with orthodox surgical treatment where cancer is concerned.

15.

TRAUMA AND RAPE

Rape is forcible sexual intercourse against the wishes of the woman. Sexual assault in all forms is on the increase, and may vary from assault on and interference with a young girl to attack and rape of an elderly woman. Physical damage may be severe, with extensive tears and bleeding from the vaginal wall, which sometimes requires surgical suturing. Bruising is common with swelling and pain, and scratches, lacerations and damage to the perineum may take some days to heal. Sexually transmitted disease is common, leading to a vaginal discharge, with Monilia or Trichomonas vaginitis especially common, and more rarely gonorrhoea and syphilis. Pregnancy is not uncommon, and generally a D&C is recommended as soon as it is diagnosed. Pregnancy can usually be prevented in rape cases by a two or three day course of a high-oestrogen contraceptive pill.

The physical effects of rape are temporary and short-lasting, but by far the greatest effect is a psychological one. Rape is always a profound shock, which may leave the woman with a great sense of anxiety and vulnerability, and often fearful and depressed.

Rape is especially damaging when it happens to the very young, who will need a great deal of specialized counselling and attention, or to the elderly, who are already feeling vulnerable. The initial reaction is usually shock, followed by anger and rage. Afterwards there may be mixed reactions of anxiety, fear and guilt, especially if the man involved is known and not a stranger, as is quite frequently the case. Loss of confidence, fear of further assaults, fear of being alone or going out, and insomnia may all be reactions which require help.

With firm support from friends and family, and especially from the family doctor, no formal psychiatric treatment is usually required. The family doctor needs to be supportive and reassuring, and to give full information about the possible risks and dangers.

The Conventional Approach to Trauma and Rape
The usual approach to rape is to deal with the physical conditions which require local treatment, especially the suturing of lacerations. When an infection is present or a possibility, then penicillin or tetracycline may be indicated. A molested child often needs specialized help and psychotherapy, and a brief period of counselling may be wise in every young case.

Recommended Remedies for Trauma and Rape

1) Aconitum
The best remedy for acute fear, shock, restless anxiety and vulnerability.

2) Arnica
Indicated for physical and psychological bruising, pain and tenderness.

3) Natrum mur.
Recommended for more long-term emotional problems with loss of confidence, fear, insomnia, and often agoraphobia.

4) Argentum nit.
When fears and phobias are very marked, together with an intolerance of heat.

5) Rescue remedy
This Bach remedy is recommended immediately after assault and for the acute period of emotional crisis following.

6) Staphisagria
For tender painful urethral or bladder bruising, and marked feelings of anger and resentment.

16.

OVARIAN DISEASE

Healthy ovarian functioning is important for the well-being of every woman. At birth the ovary contains between 100,000 and 400,000 eggs, one of which is released at ovulation time throughout the woman's menstrual life. As well as being the source of the female ovum, for a major period of adult life the ovaries produce the female hormones oestrogen and progesterone. Under direct pituitary influence, the follicle cells surrounding the ova are major hormonal producers, secreting predominantly oestrogen before the follicle cells burst to release the egg-cell at ovulation, and then from the residue of the ruptured follicle — the corpus luteum — progesterone along with oestrogen is secreted until a few days before the next period.

Ectopic Pregnancy

Fertilization and development of an egg outside the uterus occurs in about one in 300 pregnancies, or about 0.4 per cent of live births. Ectopic means 'outside' pregnancy, and in the majority of cases — 98 per cent — ectopic pregnancy means a pregnancy occurring within the fallopian tube. More rarely it may occur in the ovary itself or within the abdominal cavity. In some very rare cases an abdominal ectopic pregnancy has developed fully and the baby has survived within the abdominal cavity to be delivered safely by caesarian section, but the risks of haemorrhage are considerable, and the chances of survival of the foetus until term are extremely slim.

The fertilized egg descends through the fallopian tube into the uterus for normal embedding to occur, or fertilization may occur within the uterus. If for any reason the fertilized egg fails to descend, it becomes embedded within the fallopian tube wall, and as the primitive placenta burrows into the tube wall in search of nutrition, it usually erodes an artery and causes bleeding into the abdominal cavity with accompanying pain. In other cases the developing ovum ruptures the tube and splits it with severe pain, bleeding from the vagina, and often shock and collapse. This usually happens about the sixth week.

Causes of Ectopic Pregnancy

The commonest causes of ectopic pregnancy are previous tubal infections, especially gonorrhoea or chronic bacterial salpingitis. Congenital fallopian abnormalities are also a frequent factor, especially if the condition is recurrent, with the presence in the tube of diverticulae or blind alleyways. A growth or tumour of the tube may rarely provoke an ectopic pregnancy because of its obstruction to the normal passage of the fertilized egg into the uterus. It is also more common where a pregnancy occurs in women using an IUD contraceptive device or taking a progesterone-only contraceptive pill. Finally, an abnormal pattern of early embryonic development may provoke tubular implantation and ectopic development.

Symptoms of Ectopic Pregnancy

The usual early symptoms are that a period is delayed or 'late', followed by slight bleeding. With an ectopic pregnancy, usually only one period is missed. Vaginal bleeding often occurs after a brief period of amenorrhoea, and the loss is dark and slight, and associated with abdominal pain. The pain is characteristically severe, in the lower abdomen or referred to the shoulder, when the diaphragm is irritated by bleeding into the peritoneal cavity. The woman is pale and shocked, with a very slight rise in temperature, low blood-pressure, and the pulse weak or thready. A great deal of severe abdominal colicky pain with only slight vaginal bleeding is strongly indicative of a tubal pregnancy, and the condition can be confirmed by a positive pregnancy test.

The Conventional Approach to Ectopic Pregnancy

Because of the risks of severe haemorrhage with a risk to the woman's life, the only treatment recommended for ectopic pregnancy is immediate surgery.

Recommended Remedies for Ectopic Pregnancy

Urgent hospitalization and medical diagnosis and surgery are essential for this condition, homoeopathy playing only a secondary role in the treatment of shock until the doctor and ambulance come. Arnica and Rescue remedy may be given orally, and the woman should be kept warm and still.

Tubal Abortion

In this condition there is slight vaginal bleeding into the fallopian wall without rupture or haemorrhage, and the embryo dies in situ. It then becomes naturally dislodged and expelled by the uterus in the slight loss that occurs, perhaps after the loss or delay of one period. When the dead embryo remains in place and becomes absorbed, it is called a tubal mole, and this can sometimes be a cause of pain, infection, abdominal discomfort and an intermittent dark vaginal discharge. Tubal moles are often absorbed without further problems, but in general a diagnosed tubal mole is best removed surgically.

Pain at Ovulation

This is not an uncommon occurrence, and is thought to be related to spasm of the fallopian tubes or to a slight bleeding from the ovary at the time of ovum release which irritates the peritoneal cavity lining layer. In general it is not severe, and such measures as preventing ovulation by the use of the oral contraceptive pill are rarely required and are not to be recommended.

Recommended Remedies for Pain at Ovulation

1) Colocynth
Recommended for very severe spasms of piercing colicky pain which is often predominantly on the left side. All symptoms are better for bending double, putting firm pressure in the area, warmth and movement. The most extreme irritatability and anger is characteristic.

2) Lycopodium
I recommend this remedy for more right-sided ovarian pain, often worse in the late afternoon, less acute than described for Colocynth, and associated with a far more nervous and fearful disposition. Flatulence and indigestion are commonly present.

3) Sabina
One of the best remedies where there are violent pains, not so much spasmodic and colicky as more sustained, usually felt in the ovaries and particularly in the lower back and sacrum. The pains are always worse for heat and movement, which contrasts the remedy well with Colocynth. The

symptoms are frequently aggravated by any form of music.

4) Naja

One of the best remedies for more diffuse and generalized neuralgic pain of the left ovary, especially associated with palpitations.

Ruptured Corpus Luteum Cyst

A cause of severe abdominal pain due to excessive bleeding from over-development of the corpus luteum after ovulation. The condition needs to be differentiated carefully from an ectopic pregnancy or endometriosis. Specialized experience is necessary to make the diagnosis and a period of observation in hospital may be required to be sure that the condition does not recur. It is usually mild and does not require specific treatment.

Ovarian Cyst

This is a quite common cause of swelling without pain in the lower abdomen. The cause is generally unknown, but thought to be due to enlargement of one of the unbroken follicle cells of the ovary (called a Graffian cell) which continues to secrete fluid without an ovum being released or where an ovum has degenerated. The cyst may become as large as a grapefruit if left, and cause pressure problems on the bladder and rectum, and often pain and discomfort during sexual intercourse. If an ovarian cyst is large and causing pressure symptoms it should be removed by surgery. There is always a risk of the cyst becoming rotated so that torsion occurs with very severe pain and bleeding, which is another reason for surgical removal of a large cyst.

Recommended Remedies for Ovarian Cyst

Any pressure or obstructive condition should be treated surgically with homoeopathy in a secondary supportive role.

1) Baryta carb.

Useful for large single cystic swellings in the body generally. The woman is timid with an underdeveloped personality.

2) Calc. carb.

This remedy has often reduced cystic swellings where chilly weakness and corpulence are present with general slowness and lack of drive.

3) Graphites
Often useful for cystic conditions where sexual intercourse is painful.

4) Silicea
Recommended for chronic cystic conditions.

Endometriosis
In this condition the menstrual flow and fragments of the endometrial lining flow backwards up the fallopian tubes into the abdominal peritoneal cavity. The endometrial cells seed and survive by attaching themselves to a pelvic organ or area of tissue in the cavity, especially around the uterus and ovaries. The use of tampons is thought to be partly responsible for the condition by causing backflow and retrograde menstruation. In their new position the endometrial cells are still influenced by the output and levels of circulating oestrogen and progesterone, and during menstruation they become congested and filled with blood, and exert pressure in the area where they have seeded. With successive retrograde bleedings, the seeding areas accumulate to form large masses of engorged cystic cells, full of dark blood, which leak and cause severe pain and abdominal sensitivity and tenderness.

The Conventional Approach to Endometriosis
Surgery has been widely used in the past, but in recent years removal of the affected areas and associated neighbouring organs has been used less. Progesterone is given in an attempt to damp down the cells, usually as oral progesterone or Danol (Danazol).

Recommended Remedies for Endometriosis
There are no specific remedies recommended. Refer to the section on dysmenorrhoea (page 37) and follow the remedies which best match the symptoms, their time of occurrence, and side of the abdomen most affected.

Ovarian Cancer
Ovarian cancer affects about 1 per cent of women who have cancer, and is not very common. About 94 per cent of all ovarian swellings or tumours are benign and come into the other groups already discussed. The problem with ovarian cancer is that it is largely silent and difficult to diagnose in its early stages. Often the earliest symptoms are vague discomfort or indigestion, and perhaps a vague and variable discomfort during sexual intercourse. For many women the first real symptom is an abdominal lump

with a sense of heaviness. Sometimes an unexplained thrombophlebitis of one leg is a first warning sign. Whenever there is vague and unexplained abdominal discomfort it must be treated seriously and a careful and full examination carried out. Diagnosis may be difficult, particularly at an early stage, and is often only made by exploratory surgical operation (laparotomy) or visualization of the ovary through the abdominal cavity (laparoscopy). With early diagnosis, surgery can make a complete cure possible.

The Conventional Approach to Ovarian Cancer

The usual treatment of ovarian cancer is the removal of the affected ovary and tubes. Chemotherapy and radiotherapy may be required as adjuncts to surgery. In general it is doubtful whether the ovaries should be removed as a cancer prevention measure at the same time as a hysterectomy, although this has been routine procedure for many surgeons, and it should be a matter for personal discussion between patient and doctor. When the ovaries are removed at the time of a hysterectomy there can often be severe and unpleasant menopausal withdrawal symptoms. Pelvic ultrasound examination can now detect a slightly enlarged ovary before it can be felt clinically. This is a major new technical advance.

Recommended Remedies for Ovarian Cancer

My approach to this disease follows my general comments in the chapter on cancer. Proper and early diagnosis is vital for ovarian cancer, and the condition should be suspected whenever vague discomfort fails to respond to a seemingly well-indicated prescription. The correct course of treatment for all forms of cancer is not homoeopathy, but surgery. Homoeopathy has a role to play in the preparatory phase before an operation and during convalescence, but its role is not a primary one for this disease.

17.

CONTRACEPTION

Plants have traditionally been used as contraceptives with some success, but at present there is no effective homoeopathic 'alternative' contraceptive agent which has been satisfactorily developed. It is unlikely that this will ever happen for a variety of reasons. A contraceptive method must be at least 98 per cent consistently effective in order to be recommended and homoeopathy cannot guarantee this sort of success rate. Apart from this, homoeopathy is primarily about the treatment and prevention of symptoms and illnesses, and pregnancy is not an illness. Homoeopathy can however be helpful in the side-effects of orthodox prevention methods, which are most marked in women taking oral contraceptives.

If there is no homoeopathic pill, why is a homoeopath writing about contraception? The answer has to do with the homoeopathic approach to health. Homoeopathy is not only about prescribing, it is about an attitude to the patient which believes that prevention is at least as important as cure, and that information is vital to every patient so that they can be both better informed and in the best position to act effectively and intelligently.

It is important to recognize that all modern contraceptive knowledge is very recent, and it is only since 1940 that the role of oestrogen and progesterone as ovulation inhibitors has been known. Since that time many hormonal methods have been tried, but none is totally satisfactory from a medical point of view.

In order to understand contraception, it is also important to understand the fertilization process which you are trying to prevent from happening. For pregnancy to occur, the sperm must be healthily and actively present in the woman's uterus or fallopian tube, and make contact with a healthy egg cell which it can fertilize. Implantation or embedding within the endothelial lining of the uterus must then occur for further development of the placenta to occur healthily and safely. Sperm ejaculated outside the vagina but within the vulval area can frequently swim up inside the vagina to reach the uterus. The life of sperm within the vagina is approximately six hours, so that a mechanical contraceptive barrier must prevent sperm from uterine entry for at least that period of time after the man's orgasm, and should not be removed within six hours of intercourse. Although the intravaginal sperm life is relatively short, once it has gained access into the uterus the healthy sperm finds itself in an ideal environment, and can then survive easily for up to four days. When a safe period, non-barrier method is used, then intercourse must be avoided for four days before the anticipated time of ovulation. This can create many problems and uncertainties, especially when there is doubt about the exact date of the next ovulation.

The Oral Contraceptive Pill

There are now two major types of oral contraceptive pill on the market. The commonest is the combination pill, which contains oestrogen and progesterone in varying amounts and combinations according to which pill you are taking. In general the low oestrogen combinations are now favoured, with about 15 per cent oestrogen content. The combination pill works by inhibiting ovulation, blocking the hypothalamic follicle-stimulating action so that the ovarian follicle fails to develop and mature. This type of pill also affects the endometrial lining, causing thinning of the lining, a slowing down of the rate of ovum descent in the fallopian tubes, and thickening of the cervical mucous plug which makes it less conducive to sperm penetration. This combination acts on many different areas of the genital tract, preventing contraception at every possible level. The combination pill is usually packed in cards of twenty-one pills and taken from day five of the cycle, counting the first day of bleeding as day one. If the pill is forgotten for any reason, it should be taken within twelve hours, even if that means taking two close together.

The second type of pill is called the mini-pill or continuous pill. This is a more recent development, and is a progesterone pill which acts quite differently from the combination pill. Many consider it to be much safer, with less risks than the combined approach, especially for women over thirty. Its action is much more specific and local, keeping the endometrium thin so that implantation is less likely, and thickening the cervical mucous plug to act as a sperm barrier. Ovulation is in no way affected and occurs normally. The mini-pill is packed in cards of twenty-eight pills and must be taken daily throughout the cycle at the same time of day — ideally on waking in the morning. This method is slightly less reliable than the combined one, there is a greater incidence of ectopic pregnancy, and spotting or breakthrough mid-cycle bleeding is more common.

The pill should not be taken when breast feeding, since it may diminish the amount of milk produced, and it is likely to cross the milk barrier and gain entry to the young feeding baby, which is not desirable.

The Advantages of the Oral Contraceptive Pill

The pill is convenient, easy to use, does not create a physical barrier during sex, and is not messy. It gives many women a sense of security and relaxation, but it is not 100 per cent effective, and some women become pregnant while on the pill. If you want total certainty it must be combined with the rhythmic method, but an additional mechanical barrier method is unnecessary. Other related symptoms often improve with taking the pill, such as facial acne, painful periods and premenstrual tension. The formerly recommended 'sequential pill' has now been withdrawn as dangerous to health, and you should not be taking C-quens, Norquens, Novum SQ or Ovacon — if you are you should stop immediately and seek advice from your local doctor or clinic.

Side-effects of the Pill

Nausea and headache are common, together with weight gain due to the progesterone effect on water retention. The breasts may become heavy, tender and painful, and although in general the periods become lighter, in some cases the periods may become heavier. Vaginitis, especially thrush, is common due to the progesterone effect on the vaginal cells. Many women feel generally unwell and more nervous when on the pill, and mood changes, depression, irritability and loss of libido are common. The greatest risk is thrombophlebitis and clotting, leading to stroke or heart attack. This is more dangerous in women over thirty-five especially if the woman is smoking or where there is any family history of heart or circulatory disease. Another occasional side effect of the pill is chloasma, a discolouration of the forehead, cheeks and nasal area, causing brownish staining. Corneal irritation in contact lens users sometimes occurs, and in general there is an increased predisposition to cystitis and urinary irritation problems.

Women over thirty-five should choose a mechanical method — an IUD or diaphragm — rather than the pill. When the woman is a smoker the age limit for the pill should be thirty. The pill is also best avoided when there is a family history of circulatory disease, especially of thrombophlebitis. Severe varicose veins are also an added risk, and the pill is not recommended for varicose vein sufferers because of the increased risk of thrombophlebitis.

Hypertension, raised blood pressure or previous heart disease are also indicators that the pill should not be taken, together with epilepsy, which may be aggravated by water retention, diabetes with its increased liability to circulation and heart disease, and kidney disease, because sodium balance and water circulation is interfered with by the hormones. Where there is an existing cancer the pill is not recommended, as it may exascerbate the condition by hormonal interference.

Only take the pill if you absolutely must, and you cannot accept or arrange any other method. Take it for a maximum of five years at any one time, and then stop for a rest period of several months. In every case when it is no longer necessary, use the opportunity to stop taking the pill. In recent months the high oestrogen combination sequential pill has been withdrawn as unsafe because of increased uterine cancer risks in women using it. Always take the pill with the lowest oestrogen content available. Do keep abreast of developments in contraception and don't hesitate to stop the pill if you feel unwell, and particularly if you develop a painful vein condition in the legs. Finally, do not smoke while taking the pill, because you enormously increase the dangers and risks involved.

Withdrawal (Coitus Interruptus)
Withdrawal is perhaps the oldest and simplest of all contraceptive methods. The man withdraws the penis from the vagina just prior to ejaculation, and either does not ejaculate or prevents the fluid from entering the vagina. The essential problem with this method is that it is very unreliable, since the pre-ejaculation lubricant fluid often contains healthy sperm. Withdrawal is unpredictable, difficult to control, and can be frustrating and is psychologically unhealthy.

The Intra-uterine Device (IUD)
Also called the loop or coil, the IUD's action is not completely understood but it probably prevents implantation in the endometrial embedding layer. It is a widely-used and effective method, particularly for women who have had children. It is not totally effective, however, and pregnancy or tubal pregnancy can occur. In some cases the IUD may fall out, with the woman

not realizing it until conception has taken place.

Advantages of the IUD

The major advantage of the IUD is that the woman is not exposed to repeated doses of hormones with unknown long-term effects. In general the IUD can be left in place for long periods — up to ten years — without removal, as long as it is comfortable and not causing any adverse symptoms.

Side-effects of the IUD

The intra-uterine device is a foreign body, and some women react to it with heavy bleeding, menstrual cramps and pain. Infection is always possible, although most women do not find this a problem. Perforation of the uterus can occur, with infection, high temperature or peritonitis. Sometimes the coil falls out spontaneously within the first few weeks or months, being poorly tolerated or rejected by the uterus. A replacement may be more successful, but the rejection may be repeated. Some doctors recommend a change of coil every two to three years, but many feel that if there are no problems and symptoms a coil can be left alone for up to ten years.

When there is already a history of heavy periods or flooding the method is not advisable, and similarly where there is a history of fibroids. Where there is a problem of cramping pains and severe dysmenorrhoea the IUD is unsuitable as the problem may be aggravated. A previous history of pelvic or fallopian infection may also contraindicate the IUD.

The Dutch Cap

The cap or occlusive diaphragm is widely used, and acts as a physical barrier to sperm entering into the uterine cavity and fertilizing the ovum. In general it is effective and comfortable, with few disadvantages. It is essential, however, that it is correctly fitted, otherwise it is liable to be displaced during intercourse and move from its position over the cervix. An ill-fitting cap may also be very uncomfortable during intercourse. To be fully effective it is always essential to use a recommended spermicidal cream, which must be spread over both sides of the diaphragm before insertion.

Side-effects of the Dutch Cap

Side-effects of the cap are generally few. Some women develop an itching discomfort in the area from an allergic reaction to the rubber or to the barrier cream, and sometimes there is an increased liability to cystitis and urinary discomfort. Sometimes the man can feel the device and finds it uncomfortable, and if this happens it should be checked for size. The recommended life of a cap is one year, and it should then be thrown out and replaced. Always dry the cap carefully and inspect it for damage. Check it regularly for correct fitting, especially if it falls out or causes pain or discomfort.

The very small or cervical vault caps are not recommended, since they fall out far too easily. In general, provided that the method suits the woman, there are no disadvantages or risks to using the cap, and it is effective as long as spermicidal cream is always used.

The Sheath

The sheath — also called the condom or French letter — dates back over several centuries. In general it is a very effective method provided that it is properly used, and especially if it is combined with a spermicidal cream. The method is an obvious one; the rubber sheath acts as a complete barrier to the sperm reaching the vaginal cavity, retaining the fluid in the tip of the condom so that it is unable to reach the uterus and the ovum. The disadvantages are that it is felt by some people to be an intrusion and to spoil the spontaneity of the union. For others the feel and odour of the rubber is objectionable, and lowers the pleasure of the intercourse.

Provided they are stored in a cool place away from heat and light, condoms will remain usable for two years, and after that they should be thrown out. When buying in bulk they should always be dated clearly.

To be effective the condom must be withdrawn from the vagina before the erection subsides; if this is not done there is a risk that it will come off within the vagina and undermine the precautions taken. It is most reliable when combined with either a foam pessary or a spermicidal cream.

The Rhythm Method

The rhythm or safe period method is also not new. In this method intercourse is avoided during the time of ovulation of the female cycle. There are two major methods to consider.

The Calendar Method

In this method, only applicable to a woman with a regular cycle, ovulation is assumed to occur between the tenth and fourteenth day of the cycle, and intercourse is avoided during this time. The principle is that pregnancy is avoided because the sperm is not available for fertilization at the time of ovum-release.

The Temperature Method

Here the slight rise in body temperature is used to accurately pin-point the time of ovulation. Like the calendar method, intercourse is avoided at this time which stops pregnancy occurring. The temperature is taken daily on waking, and just before ovulation there is a slight drop in temperature followed by a rise of approximately 1°F/0.5°C at the moment of ovulation, thought to be due to a rapid outflow of progesterone which occurs at this time.

Side-effects of the Rhythm Method

When using the calendar method it is impossible to know exactly when ovulation will in fact occur, and it is far too approximate to assume that ovulation will always occur between the twelfth and fourteenth days, as in some cycles it may be as early as the tenth day or as late as the sixteenth day. These disadvantages apply for a perfectly regular twenty-eight day cycle. In fact, to be reasonably sure of effective contraception, remembering that the intra-uterine lifespan of the healthy sperm can be up to four days, it is essential to avoid intercourse from day eight of the cycle to day twenty-one. The temperature method is also not reliable, although widely used in some cultures and some countries. The major disadvantage is that it only tells you when ovulation has taken place, which may be too late, especially if intercourse has occurred within the last four days, which always makes fertilization a possibility.

I consider the rhythm method ineffective, and do not recommend it to be used as the sole contraceptive approach if you really want to avoid pregnancy. It is best combined with a spermicidal cream or foam pessary. When a period starts with a little loss or a false alarm, it becomes impossible to ascertain the exact start of the cycle, which also makes the method very unreliable. It has a high failure rate, but of course it is the most natural method with no health risk to the woman.

Spermicidal Methods

A variety of intra-vaginal chemical substances have been used, usually ineffectively, over the years, including substances such as salt — which happens to be a very effective spermicidal agent — quinine and citric acid. The modern spermicide destroys the live sperm within the vagina, and is usually in the form of a cream, paste, tablet or foam pessary. Their effective lifespan is only about one hour, so they are really only effective when applied shortly before intercourse, and they are most effective when combined with one of the mechanical methods already discussed.

Side-effects of Spermicidal Methods

To date few serious problems have arisen. The major problems are allergic irritations, rashes and reactions, with itching eczemas and sometimes a mild allergic vaginitis. In general they are not very satisfactory for the woman, since they nearly always feel messy, damp and uncomfortable, and they are very unreliable. The use of a spermicide is essential with the diaphragm, and is recommended as an adjunct to other mechanical methods.

Sterilization

Sterilization involves the surgical operation of ligation or tying of the fallopian tubes to create a permanent physical barrier. Part of each tube is usually removed so the operation cannot usually be reversed. A more recent technique is cauterization by means of an electric current, creating a total blockage by causing fibrosis of the fallopian tubes. Other techniques involve the use of clips, but this may be less reliable. Sterilization is often routinely carried out after a second or third caesarian birth in the interests of the mother's health. It is an operation without complications or after-effects.

Vasectomy

Vasectomy is the male equivalent to sterilization. The vas deferens between the testicle and penis is cut and tied, creating a permanent and irreversible blockage to sperm movement. The process does not interfere in any way with erection, ejaculation or orgasm, but the ejaculatory fluid is sterile or sperm-free. Vasectomy is a simple out-patient procedure which is highly effective and without risk. Both vasectomy and sterilization are permanent and cannot be reversed at a later date, so the couple must be totally sure that they are not going to want to become parents at a later date, either within the present relationship or any future one.

The Reliability of Contraceptive Methods

Most methods are about 95 per cent effective, and in general there is not much to chose between the reliability statistics of the various choices.

The combination oral contraceptive pill is most reliable — about 98 per cent effective.

The mini-pill or progesterone only oral contraceptive is slightly less reliable — 97 per cent effective.

The IUD is about as effective as the progesterone pill — 97 per cent effective.

The combination of a sheath and spermicidal cream or pessary foam is 98 per cent effective.

Combining the diaphragm or cap and spermicidal cream is 97 per cent effective.

The rhythmic method is optimistically recorded as 85 per cent reliable.

In the final analysis the choice of contraceptive method must be a personal one, finding a method that is as comfortable, reliable and without risk of unwanted side-effects. If your present method is uncomfortable or unsatisfactory — either physically or psychologically — do discuss it with your partner, and don't be afraid to change your method, but always do so with advice from a specialist clinic or physician.

18.

SEXUAL PROBLEMS

Painful Intercourse (Dyspareunia)

Intercourse may be painful for physical or psychological reasons. When there is a physical reason, this needs diagnosing and correcting as soon as possible in order to avoid additional emotional and psychological damage and further lack of confidence.

Physical Causes of Painful Intercourse

Local infection and soreness can make intercourse painful, especially in uncomfortable positions. Several illnesses often cause tenderness during sex, including cervical disease; ovarian disease, especially an ovarian cyst or tumour or a corpus luteum cyst; uterine disease, especially a fibroid or tumour; disease of the fallopian tubes; or endometriosis. Intercourse can often be painful after childbirth, especially too soon after an episiotomy, and vaginal dryness, especially at the menopause, can be a problem. Finally, a retroverted (malpositioned and tipped) uterus can sometimes cause discomfort during sexual intercourse.

Psychological Causes of Painful Intercourse

This is a very complicated area because there are so many possible psychological variables which cause tension and anxiety. Rushing intercourse can often cause tension and discomfort, or there may be problems of guilt, immaturity, or ambivalence and hostility towards the partner. In many cases spasm and tension in the genital region are primarily of emotional origin, and the problem needs clearing by discussion and understanding between the couple. Enough time must be allowed for the woman to respond and relax.

Recommended Remedies for Painful Intercourse

a) Where the cause is physical

1) Hepar sulph.
For simple local infective conditions.

2) Nitric acid
Where there is a crack, tear or fissure causing severe burning discomfort.

3) Silicea
Where there is a long-standing local painful infection, sometimes with a purulent discharge. Silicea is also suitable for a local boil or abscess.

b) Where the cause is psychological

1) Ammonium carb.
The pain is felt deeply in the vaginal vault, cervix or uterus, the discomfort worse before and during a period.

2) Belladonna
Where there is pain with dryness, and the most extreme sensitivity to touch or sudden movements. Burning discomfort is often typical. Belladonna is usually best for more recent problems.

3) Bryonia
There is dryness but without the great sensitivity of Belladonna. There is a general absence of moisture and lubrication, often with obstinate constipation.

4) Lycopodium
The skin is dry, the vagina is sore and lacks lubrication, and the woman is anxious, miserable and lacking in confidence. She is over-sensitive, gives up easily, and easily feels a complete failure. Indigestion is frequent.

5) Natrum mur.
Dryness is marked, but there is a deep-seated psychological problem which causes tension, tears, and sometimes aversion.

6) Staphisagria
There is pain with lancing severity, irritability, oversensitivity, sexuality often heightened.

7) Thuja
A combination of dryness, irritability, extreme sensitivity, and immature sexuality.

Loss of Libidinal Interest

This is nearly always a psychological problem, although it can often be associated with and exacerbated by fatigue, anaemia, the pill, and a whole variety of exhausting physical circumstances. Variation in the level of libidinal interest is normal, and often varies within the female cycle. Libido may diminish during pregnancy, at the menopause, when there is a problem of premenstrual tension, or due to various diseases including diabetes, anaemia, obesity, alcoholism, herpes or vaginitis. In the main, however, these circumstances usually only exaggerate an already existing psychological problem.

Recommended Remedies for Loss of Libido

1) Agnus cast.
One of the most useful remedies where there is marked feebleness, exhaustion, and overall loss of energy and drive. Depression is nearly always marked, with fatigue and lack of vitality and libido, usually with aversion to the opposite sex.

2) Ammonium carbonate
There is a long-standing and intransigent thick, whitish and often excoriating vaginal discharge. This is combined with an irritating painful vulval condition and lack of libido and aversion to intercourse.

3) Onosmodium
This is sometimes recommended, but I suggest it only as a back-up remedy to the more deeply-acting remedies.

4) Sepia
One of the best remedies where there is indifference, lack of libido, irritability, fatigue, dragging pains and exhaustion, always better for brisk walking,

exercise or dancing. Constipation and hunger are marked.

5) *Silicea*

There is general weakness and lack of drive or initiative. Frequently there are tender, painful areas of cracking, fissure or discharge, often with a purulent loss. Chilliness and sweating are marked.

Frigidity

The inability to achieve orgasm in intercourse is always of psychological origin. It is difficult to assess its frequency, but it is a very common and often hidden problem which is not sufficiently discussed either with the woman's doctor, or for that matter with the partner. Both measures would usually go some way towards inproving the situation.

Causes of Frigidity

A major reason for frigidity is a lack of knowledge and information about sexual matters, and not just about intercourse. Frigidity is often a reflection of unresolved sexual conflicts, often early and infantile in origin, and chronic tension between the couple and failure to be sufficiently open and honest can cause frigidity. The fear of loss of control in orgasm is probably a very common problem, and is often linked with a tendency to be over-controlled in everything. Lack of confidence is frequently associated, but is often well hidden by social skills, so that it may not always be obvious to anyone except the individual woman and her partner. Fatigue, convalescence and physical illness are rarer causes.

Frigidity is a frequent and distressing problem. There is usually no problem at all in achieving a masturbatory orgasm; it is only with the man that orgasm does not occur, which often creates the most intense feelings of irritability, failure and depression. In general there is no loss of libidinal sexual interest, and it may even be heightened.

An important point to remember is that no woman experiences orgasm every time. Each experience of sexual intercourse is a unique event, different in the quality of feelings and orgasm. Often a woman does experience multiple orgasms during sexual act, contrasting with the single masculine orgasm, but it is perfectly normal not to have orgasms for a period of several weeks or even months. Only if the problem lasts for many months should you consider getting help.

Recommended Remedies for Frigidity

1) Agnus cast.
One of the best remedies, provided that the typical weakness and exhaustion are present.

2) Nat. mur.
Useful when there is a combination of dryness and marked psychological factors. The woman is usually a 'loner' and tends to tearful depression.

3) Phosphorus
One of the best and deepest acting remedies. The woman is popular, social and outgoing, although rather timid. Sexual interest and desire is marked and vigorous, but in spite of a great deal of effort and physical involvement, the vagina persists in feeling swollen or sore, sometimes with a slight bleeding, and orgasm remains unattainable. Frustration, nervousness and depression with tears are often related to the sense of failure. The libido often does not subside after intercourse.

4) Sepia
One of the best remedies where there is irritability, exhaustion, constipation and general indifference alongside the loss of libidinal interest. The woman only wants to eat and then rest and sleep. Low back ache is often constant and chronic.

5) Silicea
Useful after Sepia where there is general weakness, low libidinal drive, and absent orgasm. Chilliness with sweating and pallor is frequent, and the woman is thin and underweight.

Spasm and Vaginismus
The involuntary spasm and contraction of the vaginal muscles, preventing intercourse, is fairly rare, but can be a problem. The condition is accompanied by the most extreme sensitivity of the vulval-vaginal region, which at the least physical contact goes into tight spasm, preventing even the introduction of a tampon or cap, and often preventing physical examination by a doctor. The cause of vaginismus is nearly always psychological, and is often associated with an oversensitive or volatile disposition, and underlying fear and lack of confidence. More rarely, there is a tight, non-yielding hymen,

or a minute painful crack in the region of the vaginal entrance.

Treatments for vaginismus include specialized counselling techniques, self-examination, and exploration, often involving the partner in a process of slowly desensitizing the vagina. Glass dilators are sometimes recommended to overcome the spasm.

Recommended Remedies for Spasm or Vaginismus

1) *Actea racemosa (Cimicifugea racemosa)*
One of the most useful remedies for problems of vaginal and uterine spasm and contraction. The woman is always freezing cold, and warmth helps all the symptoms of this remedy. The psychological make-up is hysterical and very varied and changeable, resembling Pulsatilla, but the latter is aggravated by the least warmth or heat.

2) *Belladonna*
Useful where the spasm is hot and burning, and there is associated restlessness with intolerance of touch or movement.

3) *Cactus grand.*
Often a useful remedy where the spasm is severe, and cardiac symptoms or palpitations are associated.

4) *Coffea*
Consider this remedy where the vaginal spasm is associated with marked nervousness, restlessness, irritability and insomnia.

5) *Kreosotum*
Often recommended, especially where there is an associated thick offensive vaginal discharge and irritability is marked.

6) *Platina*
An important remedy when the typical haughty superior Platina temperament is in evidence.

7) *Plumbum*
Probably the best remedy to consider for obstinate and severe vaginal spasm. Constipation is always severe.

8) Thuja
This is a very deep acting remedy and is indicated where there is severe chronic spasm, marked sweating, and often strange ideas about sexuality and the body image generally.

Anxiety and Fear of Sexual Intercourse

This is a common problem, which often occurs as a result of lack of knowledge about sex. As they grew up, many women were led to believe that sexuality and sexual fantasies were wrong, bad and dirty. In this environment the natural expression of libido has become laden with guilt, conflict, repression and denial.

The psychological preparation for relaxed and enjoyable adult intercourse begins in childhood, and from the earliest stages of youthful awareness of pleasure and comfort. In these early years there is a quite normal interest in genital exploration and pleasure, and a great deal of curiosity about the body and its orifices and openings, especially the pleasurable and erotic areas. In a healthy family such curiosity is seen and understood as part of normal growth, and not implying that the child has bad habits. In this way sex does not have to become something naughty, secret or dirty, but just a natural part of how we feel and express ourselves.

When there is parental ease and relaxation, sexuality does not become a matter of anxiety or fear, but something increasingly sensitive and important, and a way of expressing affection, closeness and tenderness. As well as being a way of expressing closeness between people, sexuality is also part of the way in which we can appreciate our own bodies. Masturbation is often a major area of misplaced concern in an unhealthy or immature family and can all too easily become a thing of shame and guilt. The reality is that masturbation is normal, harmless and ubiquitous. It is often an important need at certain times of life, and most of all it is pleasurable, a physical outlet and a relief from tension in many cases. It is only harmful when associated with the negative tags of guilt and shame.

The Conventional Approach to Anxiety and Fear of Sexual Intercourse

In a modern enlightened clinic, information and reassurance are freely given, with specialized psychotherapy or counselling being made available. Try and avoid the use of tranquillizers or sedatives if possible; they only serve to dampen or further reduce normal libidinal levels. They are also strongly addictive, and when you want to come off them you may find that you have the additional problem of drug dependency.

Recommended Remedies for Anxiety and Fear of Sexual Intercourse

1) *Argentum nit.*
I recommend this remedy where there is extreme phobic anxiety, fear and often panic, together with the most intense intolerance of heat of any form.

2) *Ignatia*
I use this remedy where this is either a severe hysterical problem, or wherever grief and loss are associated.

3) *Lycopodium*
A useful and deep acting psychological remedy for insecurity hidden beneath a cloak of intellect and apparent maturity. There is charm and social aplomb, but fear and insecurity lie beneath.

4) *Pulsatilla*
One of the best female sexual remedies where the problem is of flirtation and provocation followed by tears, denial and flight. Heat is not tolerated and there is an absence of thirst.

5) *Sulphur*
Recommended for chronic problems which are not responding well to other remedies.

Excessive Desire

Excessive female desire, sometimes called nymphomania, is very much a matter of definition, and usually male definition. Such a condition is hardly ever seen clinically. In general it is a male problem, and is more likely to be complained about by a repressed and frightened man than by a woman.

Sexual desire varies enormously, and it is pointless to try to define a normal level of desire. Only when sexuality becomes uncomfortable and out of control should it become a matter for concern for the woman, and the diagnosis of any apparent problem should be made by her and not by a man. When in doubt ask for advice; if you think it is not a strictly medical problem, then discuss it first with a friend.

Excessive sexual desire is a completely relative term, and a high libidinal drive is very healthy and generally no longer considered to be abnormal. It is all a matter of individual physical and psychological well-being, and it is hardly ever a psychological problem or a matter for medical treatment. It is more a question of maturing social attitudes, and although we have already made a lot of headway, there is still room for a lot more progress to be made before such problems will be finally laid to rest.

As with excessive desire, excessive masturbation is difficult to define because the norms are so vague and vary so much with the individual. All you can do is to ask yourself whether there is an obsessional or compulsive element to your repetitive needs. If there is an overwhelming need to achieve orgasm over and over again, with increased anxiety and little fulfillment or satisfaction, then there may be an obsessional problem which needs professional advice and help from a sensitive counsellor or therapist. In addition, homoeopathic remedies are frequently very effective in helping to breakdown the power of such compulsions.

Recommended Remedies for Excessive Desire

1) Lachesis
A useful deep-acting remedy for excessive sexual excitement, often uncontrollable, and most marked after sleep. Jealousy is a characteristic emotion, which can be violent.

2) Lilium tig.
Libido is markedly heightened, with spasms of depression and violent irritability.

3) Murex
This resembles Sepia in many ways, especially with symptoms of low back pain and abdominal discomfort, exhaustion and constipation, but it is particularly indicated by heightened sexual anxiety.

4) Platina
One of the most useful remedies where treatment is required. Here there is the most extreme sensitivity of the whole vaginal and vulval region, spasm to the point of vaginismus, and aggravation during pregnancy. The disposition is one of haughty pride, with a superiority that hides feelings of insecurity and vulnerability.

5) Staphisgria
Useful where there is an uncontrollable libidinal drive, painful lancing spasms, and moodiness with irritability and resentment.

6) Zincum
Indicated where there is great excitement and restlessness, worse at night.

Premature Ejaculation
This is a common male problem, where ejaculation occurs too soon, and long before the woman has reached the height of her arousal. The man is over-excited and too sensitive, and ejaculation often occurs immediately on vaginal penetration or even before, followed by the loss of his erection. It is frequent in anxious, inexperienced men, or where the woman takes more sexual initiative. The cause is always a psychological one, and usually is not a physical problem. The man is often unsure of himself, especially in the company of women. He often feels insecure or inadequate concerning it and will often avoid a relationship because of it, yet at the same time he is usually unable or unwilling to discuss it with his partner or with his doctor, and often it is the woman who takes the initiative in organizing a consultation and possible treatment.

The Conventional Approach to Premature Ejaculation
The usual approach is professional counselling with a trained sex therapist, or a brief period of psychotherapy is advised. The Masters and Johnson technique is giving good results, and should be given by an experienced trained practitioner.

Recommended Remedies for Premature Ejaculation

1) Causticum
This is often helpful, especially where there is any associated pain with the orgasm, and ejaculation, spasm or over-control.

2) Lycopodium
I regard this as one of the best of all remedies where there is nervousness and lack of confidence. There is a general tendency to procrastination in a man with an intellectual temperament, who is otherwise caring, sensitive and attentive.

3) Medorrhinum
I strongly recommend this remedy for the type of man who is always in a hurry with every aspect of life and living. He is impatient with everything, not just with sex. Often he cannot see or admit this, and the diagnosis may have to rest with the woman to ensure accuracy.

Impotence
Impotence is the failure in a man to achieve an erection capable of penetrating the vaginal cavity, often associated with delayed or absent ejaculation. Like its female counterpart of frigidity, it is nearly always psychological in origin. The commonest physical causes of impotence include fatigue, alcohol and drugs. Impotence can also be induced by illness such as anaemia, diabetes, heart disease, arthritis and mumps, the latter often causing testicular involvement of the adult male.

However important the physical causes, it is important to recognize that this is primarily a psychological problem where insecurity is the major difficulty. Not uncommonly there is a lot of anger and resentment under the surface, and work or social problems like retirement, redundancy, job insecurity or difficult work relationships can only add to existing fears about adequacy and performance.

Impotence is divided into two major groups for convenience of diagnosis and treatment. Primary impotence is where there is total lack of erection, and penetration has never been achieved. Primary impotence is rare. Secondary impotence is where there has been an obvious precipitating cause such as a heart attack, a prostatectomy, shock, loss or trauma.

The Conventional Approach to Impotence
Primary impotence is usually treated by hormone replacements. Secondary impotence is treated by a remedy for the cause. When there is an underlying and untreated diabetes, anaemia or fatigue, this must naturally be remedied first of all. In a modern clinic or centre physical treatment is followed by discussion or counselling. Psychotherapy may be recommended, and acupuncture may be recommended as an alternative approach which may sometimes be effectively combined with homoeopathy.

Recommended Remedies for Impotence

1) Agnus cast.
One of the most effective remedies where there is weakness, exhaustion, chill, lack of vitality and drive.

2) *Bufo*
Often of value where there is a problem of primary impotence.

3) *Caladium*
Here there is strong desire but lack of an erection. Genital pruritus or itching is frequently present as an additional problem.

4) *Calc. carb.*
Symptoms include chilly weakness, a lack of power and interest, and a tendency to obesity.

5) *Cuprum met.*
Often indicated where genital spasm or cramps are present with an erection which is weak or spasmodic.

6) *Sabal serr.*
One of the most useful remedies for secondary impotence, where there is desire and interest, but weak or barely adequate erections.

7) *Selenium*
This is often recommended for weakness of erections.

A Demanding or Insensitive Partner
This is a common problem which should be dealt with by open discussion, perferably away from the bedroom, where it may do harm if discussed too close to an already delicate situation. Make sure there is enough time, for this is a topic of such importance that it should not be rushed or put off again until later. Try and explain your feelings, and exactly when and how you feel under pressure from him or are unable to respond. Try not to complain or blame, but be positive and loving in putting over your problem, and try to admit areas where you feel you have been equally demanding and insensitive. Attempt to see the process as one of joint growth within your relationship whatever the problems.

You will both need to be as sensitive as possible, and listen attentively and carefully to what the other says in reply. Try and understand how your partner sees you, and don't be too intellectual or analytical. It is often helpful to leave time after the discussion for intercourse, especially when you feel you may have made a communications breakthrough.

It is difficult to recommend a remedy because of all the variables, but I suggest only one remedy which may be helpful.

Nux vom.
This is a useful remedy for men where there is a combination of insensitivity and irritability in an otherwise sensitive man with great depths. He is often intolerant of others and their faults, and is sometimes unpopular and feels misunderstood by others.

LIST OF
RECOMMENDED REMEDIES

Aconitum
Actea race.
Agnus cast.
Aletris far.
Alumina
Ambra grisea
Ammon. carb.
Amyl nitrite
Ant. tart.
Apis
Arg. nit.
Arnica
Arsen. alb.
Asafoetida
Atropine
Aurum met.
Baryta carb.
Belladonna
Berberis
Bryonia
Bufo
Cactus grand.
Calendula
Calcarea
Calc. iod.

Cantharis
Carbo animalis
Carbo veg.
Causticum
Chelidonium
China
Colocynthis
Coffea
Conium
Crocus sat.
Crotalus
Cuprum met.
Dulcamara
Ferrum met.
Ferrum phos.
Fraxinus Amer.
Graphites
Hepar sulph.
Hyoscyamus
Ignatia
Iodium
Ipecacuanha
Kali. carb.
Kreosotum
Lachesis

Lapis alb.
Lilium tig.
Lycopodium
Mag. phos.
Medorrhinum
Mercurius
Murex
Naja
Natrum mur.
Nitric acid
Nux vom.
Onosmodium
Opium
Petroleum
Phellandrium
Phosphorus
Phosphoric acid
Phytolacca
Phytolacca berry
Psorinum
Pulsatilla
Rescue remedy (Bach
  remedy)
Rhus tox.
Sabal serrulata

Sabina	*Staphisagria*	*Thuja*
Scilla	*Stramonium*	*Thyrodinum*
Secale	*Sulphur*	*Tuberculinum bov.*
Selenium	*Tabacum*	*Urtica*
Sepia	*Tarentula hisp.*	*Veratrum alb.*
Silicea	*Terebinth*	*Zincum met.*

Homeopathic Organizations

Each of the following organizations was founded to promote the study and practice of homeopathy in the United States. These groups, comprised of physicians, adjunct health care professionals, and lay people, provide beginning, intermediate, and advanced training in homeopathy to lay people and health professionals; publish monthly or quarterly newsletters or journals; and provide many other valuable services and information.

Foundation for Homeopathic
Education and Research
2124 Kittredge Street
Berkeley, CA 94704
510-649-8930

International Foundation for
Homeopathy
2366 Eastlake Avenue E. #329
Seattle, WA 98102
206-324-8230

Homeopathic Educational Services
2124 Kittredge Street
Berkeley, CA 94704
510-649-0294

National Center for Homeopathy
801 North Fairfax Street
Suite 306
Arlington, VA 22314
703-548-7790

Suppliers of Homeopathic Remedies and Books

Biological Homeopathic Industries, Inc.
11600 Cochiti Southeast
Albuquerque, NM 87123
1-800-621-7644

Boericke and Tafel, Inc.
2381 Circadian Way
Santa Rosa, CA 95407
1-800-272-2820
1-800-876-9505

Boiron
1208 Amosland Road
Norwood, PA 19074
1-800-258-8823

INDEX